EPI DIET COOKBOOK

AND FOOD LIST

FOR BEGINNERS

Delicious Recipes and Nutritious Food for

Exocrine Pancreatic Insufficiency

Elsie A. Catanzaro

Copyright © 2024

All Rights Are Reserved

The content in this book may not be reproduced, duplicated, or transferred without the express written permission of the author or publisher. Under no circumstances will the publisher or author be held liable or legally responsible for any losses, expenditures, or damages incurred directly or indirectly as a consequence of the information included in this book.

Legal Remarks

Copyright protection applies to this publication. It is only intended for personal use. No piece of this work may be modified, distributed, sold, quoted, or paraphrased without the author's or publisher's consent.

Disclaimer Statement

Please keep in mind that the contents of this booklet are meant for educational and recreational purposes. Every effort has been made to offer accurate, up-to-date, reliable, and thorough information. There are, however, no stated or implied assurances of any kind. Readers understand that the author is providing competent counsel. The content in this book originates from several sources. Please seek the opinion of a competent professional before using any of the tactics outlined in this book. By reading this book, the reader agrees that the author will not be held accountable for any direct or indirect damages resulting from the use of the information contained therein, including, but not limited to, errors, omissions, or inaccuracies.

TABLE OF CONTENTS

INTRODUCTION

Welcome to the journey towards a healthier, happier you with the EPI Diet Cookbook and Food List for Beginners! If you're reading this, chances are you've been recently diagnosed with Exocrine Pancreatic Insufficiency (EPI), and you're feeling a whirlwind of emotions – confusion, frustration, maybe even a little fear. Trust me, I get it.

Navigating life with EPI can feel like embarking on an uncertain adventure without a map. Suddenly, every meal becomes a puzzle, every bite a potential source of discomfort. But here's the thing – you're not alone, and you're certainly not without options.

This book is your compass, your guide through the world of EPI-friendly eating. Consider it your friendly companion, here to demystify the complexities of managing EPI through diet. Whether you're completely new to the EPI scene or you've been on this journey for a while, this book is designed with you in mind – to educate, inspire, and empower you to take control of your health one delicious meal at a time.

Throughout these pages, we'll dive deep into understanding what EPI is, why diet plays a crucial role in managing it, and most importantly, how you can embrace a diet that nourishes your body without sacrificing flavor or enjoyment. From stocking your pantry with EPI-friendly essentials to whipping up mouthwatering meals that satisfy both your taste buds and your nutritional needs, we've got you covered.

But more than just recipes and food lists, this book is about building a community of support and encouragement. It's about recognizing that while EPI may present its challenges, it doesn't define who you are or what you're capable of achieving. Together, we'll celebrate the victories – big and small – and navigate the setbacks with resilience and grace

CHAPTER ONE

UNDERSTANDING EPI (EXOCRINE PANCREATIC INSUFFICIENCY)

What is EPI?

Exocrine Pancreatic Insufficiency (EPI) is a condition that affects the pancreas, a vital organ responsible for producing enzymes that aid in the digestion of food. To grasp the significance of EPI, it's essential to understand the role of the pancreas in the digestive process.

The pancreas secretes enzymes such as amylase, lipase, and protease, which are crucial for breaking down carbohydrates, fats, and proteins in the food we consume. In individuals with EPI, the pancreas fails to produce a sufficient amount of these enzymes, leading to difficulties in digesting food properly.

Causes and Symptoms

EPI can be caused by various factors, with the most common being chronic pancreatitis, cystic fibrosis, pancreatic cancer, and pancreatic surgery. Chronic pancreatitis, characterized by inflammation of the pancreas over time, can lead to damage to the pancreatic tissue, impairing its ability to produce enzymes effectively.

Cystic fibrosis, a genetic disorder, affects the production of mucus, resulting in blockages in the pancreatic ducts and preventing enzymes from reaching the digestive tract. Pancreatic cancer can also obstruct the pancreatic ducts, hindering enzyme secretion. Additionally, surgical procedures involving the pancreas can sometimes lead to EPI if a significant portion of the organ is removed or damaged.

The symptoms of EPI can vary depending on the severity of the condition but often include abdominal pain, bloating, diarrhoea, weight loss, and nutritional deficiencies. Since EPI impairs the body's ability to absorb nutrients from food, individuals may experience fatigue, weakness, and vitamin deficiencies over time.

Importance of Diet in Managing EPI

Diet plays a crucial role in managing EPI and alleviating its symptoms. By making strategic dietary modifications, individuals with EPI can optimize their nutrient intake and improve their overall quality of life.

Here are some key dietary considerations for managing EPI:

1. **Enzyme Replacement Therapy (ERT)**: One of the cornerstone treatments for EPI is enzyme replacement therapy. This involves taking synthetic pancreatic enzymes with meals to aid in the digestion of food. These enzymes help compensate for the deficiency in natural pancreatic enzymes, allowing for better nutrient absorption and reducing digestive symptoms.

2. **Low-Fat Diet**: Since individuals with EPI may have difficulty digesting fats, following a low-fat diet can help minimize digestive discomfort. Foods high in saturated and trans fats, such as fried foods, fatty meats, and full-fat dairy products, should be limited or avoided. Instead, focus on lean proteins, whole grains, and healthy fats from sources like nuts, seeds, and avocados.

3. **Small, Frequent Meals**: Eating smaller, more frequent meals throughout the day can ease the burden on the digestive system and help prevent symptoms such as bloating and abdominal pain. Breaking meals down into smaller portions allows for better enzyme utilization and absorption of nutrients.

4. **High-Protein Foods**: Protein is essential for tissue repair and muscle maintenance, especially for individuals with EPI who may experience weight loss and muscle wasting. Incorporating high-protein foods such as lean meats, poultry, fish, eggs, tofu, and legumes into meals can help meet protein requirements and support overall health.

5. **Hydration**: Adequate hydration is vital for maintaining digestive health and preventing constipation, a common issue for individuals with EPI. Drinking plenty of water throughout the day can help soften stools and promote regular bowel movements. Limiting caffeinated and

alcoholic beverages, which can exacerbate dehydration, is also advisable.

6. **Supplementation**: In addition to enzyme replacement therapy, individuals with EPI may require supplementation with vitamins and minerals, particularly fat-soluble vitamins (A, D, E, and K) that are poorly absorbed due to impaired fat digestion. Working with a healthcare professional to determine appropriate supplementation is essential to prevent nutrient deficiencies and support overall health.

7. **Fiber-Rich Foods**: Including fibre-rich foods such as fruits, vegetables, whole grains, and legumes in the diet can help promote regularity and prevent constipation. However, individuals with EPI should be mindful of high-fibre foods that may exacerbate digestive symptoms and adjust their intake accordingly.

8. **Avoiding Trigger Foods**: Certain foods and beverages can exacerbate digestive symptoms in individuals with EPI. Common triggers include spicy foods, caffeine, alcohol, and high-fat or greasy foods. Identifying and avoiding these trigger foods can help minimize discomfort and improve digestive function.

CHAPTER TWO

OVERVIEW OF THE EPI DIET

Principles and Goals

When it comes to managing Exocrine Pancreatic Insufficiency (EPI) through diet, several key principles and goals guide individuals in making informed dietary choices to optimize their nutritional intake and minimize digestive discomfort. Let's delve into these principles and goals in detail:

1. **Balanced Nutrition**: The primary goal of the EPI diet is to ensure that individuals receive adequate nutrition despite the challenges posed by impaired pancreatic enzyme production. This involves consuming a balanced diet that provides essential nutrients such as proteins, carbohydrates, fats, vitamins, and minerals in the right proportions to support overall health and well-being.

2. **Optimizing Digestion**: One of the main principles of the EPI diet is to facilitate the digestion and absorption of nutrients by minimizing the workload on the pancreas. This often involves making dietary modifications to compensate for the insufficient production of pancreatic enzymes. By choosing easily digestible foods and adopting cooking methods that break down food more effectively, individuals

can improve nutrient absorption and reduce digestive symptoms.

3. **Managing Symptoms**: Another crucial aspect of the EPI diet is managing symptoms such as abdominal pain, bloating, diarrhea, and weight loss. This may entail identifying trigger foods that exacerbate symptoms and avoiding or limiting their intake. Additionally, individuals may benefit from eating smaller, more frequent meals to ease the burden on the digestive system and prevent discomfort.

4. **Preventing Nutritional Deficiencies**: Individuals with EPI are at an increased risk of developing nutritional deficiencies due to impaired nutrient absorption. Therefore, a key goal of the EPI diet is to prevent deficiencies in essential nutrients such as fat-soluble vitamins (A, D, E, and K), as well as protein, calcium, and iron. This often requires supplementation and/or careful dietary planning to ensure adequate nutrient intake.

5. **Promoting Healthy Weight Maintenance**: Weight loss and malnutrition are common challenges for individuals with EPI, necessitating a focus on maintaining a healthy weight and preventing muscle wasting. This may involve consuming calorie-dense foods and incorporating high-protein sources into meals to support muscle mass and energy levels.

6. **Enhancing Quality of Life**: Ultimately, the overarching goal of the EPI diet is to enhance the quality of life for individuals living with the condition. By providing practical dietary guidelines and strategies for managing symptoms, the EPI diet aims to empower individuals to take control of their health and well-being, enabling them to enjoy a fulfilling and satisfying lifestyle.

In summary, the principles and goals of the EPI diet revolve around achieving optimal nutrition, optimizing digestion, managing symptoms, preventing nutritional deficiencies, promoting healthy weight maintenance, and enhancing overall quality of life for individuals with EPI. By adhering to these principles and goals, individuals can effectively manage their condition and lead fulfilling lives.

Foods to Include and Avoid

Choosing the right foods is crucial for individuals with Exocrine Pancreatic Insufficiency (EPI) to support optimal digestion, prevent symptoms, and maintain overall health. Here's a comprehensive guide to the foods to include and avoid in an EPI-friendly diet:

Foods to Include:

1. **Lean Proteins**: Incorporate lean sources of protein into your diet, such as poultry (chicken, turkey), fish, lean cuts of beef or pork, tofu, and legumes (beans, lentils). These foods provide essential amino acids for muscle maintenance

and repair without excessive fat content that may be difficult to digest.

2. **Complex Carbohydrates**: Choose complex carbohydrates that are high in fiber and nutrients, such as whole grains (brown rice, quinoa, oats), fruits, vegetables, and legumes. These foods provide sustained energy and promote digestive health by supporting regular bowel movements.

3. **Healthy Fats**: Include small amounts of healthy fats in your diet from sources such as avocados, nuts, seeds, and olive oil. These fats are rich in monounsaturated and polyunsaturated fats, which are beneficial for heart health and can be easier to digest compared to saturated and trans fats.

4. **Low-Lactose Dairy**: Opt for low-lactose or lactose-free dairy products, such as lactose-free milk, yogurt, and cheese, if tolerated. These dairy alternatives provide calcium and vitamin D for bone health without exacerbating digestive symptoms associated with lactose intolerance.

5. **Enzyme-Rich Foods**: Incorporate enzyme-rich foods into your diet to support digestion, such as pineapple, papaya, kiwi, and fermented foods like yogurt, kefir, and sauerkraut. These foods contain natural enzymes that can aid in the breakdown of nutrients and ease digestive discomfort.

6. **Hydrating Foods**: Choose hydrating foods with high water content, such as cucumbers, tomatoes, watermelon, and broth-based soups, to prevent dehydration and promote regularity. Staying hydrated is essential for maintaining digestive health and preventing constipation.

7. **Nutrient-Dense Foods**: Focus on nutrient-dense foods that provide a wide range of vitamins and minerals to support overall health and well-being. Include a variety of colorful fruits and vegetables, nuts, seeds, and whole grains in your diet to ensure adequate nutrient intake.

Foods to Avoid or Limit:

1. **High-Fat Foods**: Avoid or limit high-fat foods that may be difficult to digest, such as fried foods, fatty meats, creamy sauces, and rich desserts. These foods can exacerbate symptoms of EPI and lead to discomfort, bloating, and diarrhea.

2. **High-Lactose Dairy**: Limit or avoid high-lactose dairy products if you experience lactose intolerance symptoms, such as gas, bloating, and diarrhea. These products include regular milk, ice cream, and soft cheeses that contain significant amounts of lactose.

3. **Processed and Spicy Foods**: Minimize intake of processed foods, spicy foods, and condiments that may irritate the digestive tract and trigger symptoms such as heartburn,

indigestion, and acid reflux. Opt for homemade meals prepared with fresh, whole ingredients whenever possible.

4. **High-Sugar Foods**: Reduce consumption of high-sugar foods and beverages, such as sugary snacks, desserts, sodas, and fruit juices, which can contribute to fluctuations in blood sugar levels and exacerbate digestive symptoms. Choose natural sweeteners like honey or maple syrup in moderation.

5. **Gas-Producing Foods**: Limit intake of gas-producing foods that may cause bloating and discomfort, such as beans, broccoli, cabbage, onions, and carbonated beverages. These foods can exacerbate digestive symptoms and contribute to intestinal gas buildup.

6. **Alcohol and Caffeine**: Restrict or avoid alcohol and caffeine, which can irritate the digestive tract and lead to dehydration. These substances can worsen symptoms of EPI, such as abdominal pain, diarrhea, and nutrient malabsorption.

In summary, following an EPI-friendly diet involves including nutrient-dense foods that support digestion and overall health while avoiding or limiting foods that may exacerbate symptoms and impair nutrient absorption. By making thoughtful dietary choices and listening to your body's cues, you can effectively manage EPI and enjoy a satisfying and nourishing diet.

Importance of Enzyme Replacement Therapy (ERT)

Enzyme Replacement Therapy (ERT) is a cornerstone treatment for individuals with Exocrine Pancreatic Insufficiency (EPI) and plays a crucial role in supporting digestion, nutrient absorption, and overall health. Let's explore the importance of ERT in managing EPI and its benefits for individuals living with the condition:

1. **Compensating for Pancreatic Insufficiency**: The primary function of ERT is to compensate for the insufficient production of pancreatic enzymes in individuals with EPI. By taking supplemental pancreatic enzymes with meals and snacks, individuals can enhance the breakdown and absorption of nutrients from food, thereby alleviating symptoms and improving nutritional status.

2. **Improving Digestive Function**: ERT helps to optimize digestive function by providing the enzymes necessary for the breakdown of carbohydrates, fats, and proteins in the diet. This enables individuals with EPI to more effectively digest and absorb nutrients, reducing symptoms such as bloating, abdominal pain, diarrhea, and weight loss.

3. **Supporting Nutrient Absorption**: Proper digestion and absorption of nutrients are essential for maintaining overall health and preventing nutritional deficiencies in individuals with EPI. ERT facilitates the absorption of essential nutrients such as fat-soluble vitamins (A, D, E, and K),

protein, calcium, and iron, which may be poorly absorbed due to pancreatic insufficiency.

4. **Promoting Weight Maintenance and Muscle Health**: EPI can lead to weight loss and muscle wasting due to malabsorption of nutrients and impaired digestion. By improving nutrient absorption and supporting digestive function, ERT helps individuals with EPI maintain a healthy weight and preserve muscle mass, thereby improving energy levels and overall well-being.

5. **Enhancing Quality of Life**: Effective management of EPI with ERT can significantly enhance the quality of life for individuals living with the condition. By reducing symptoms, improving nutritional status, and supporting overall digestive health, ERT enables individuals to enjoy a more active, fulfilling lifestyle without the limitations imposed by EPI-related symptoms.

6. **Tailored Treatment Approach**: ERT is available in various formulations, including pancreatic enzyme capsules, tablets, and powders, allowing for a tailored treatment approach based on individual needs and preferences. Healthcare providers can work with patients to adjust dosage, timing, and formulation of ERT to optimize efficacy and minimize side effects.

7. **Long-Term Management**: ERT is typically a lifelong treatment for individuals with EPI, requiring ongoing

adherence to ensure optimal digestive function and nutritional status. Regular monitoring by healthcare providers is essential to assess treatment efficacy, adjust dosage as needed, and address any concerns or complications that may arise.

CHAPTER THREE

ESSENTIAL NUTRIENTS FOR EPI PATIENTS

Proteins, Fats, and Carbohydrates

Proteins, fats, and carbohydrates are the three macronutrients essential for maintaining optimal health and providing the body with energy. Each macronutrient serves unique roles in the body and plays a crucial part in supporting various physiological functions.

Let's explore the importance of proteins, fats, and carbohydrates in the diet:

Proteins:

Proteins are often referred to as the building blocks of life, and for good reason. They are essential for the growth, repair, and maintenance of tissues, muscles, organs, and cells throughout the body. Proteins are made up of amino acids, which are the basic structural units that combine to form different proteins.

In the context of managing Exocrine Pancreatic Insufficiency (EPI), protein plays a vital role in supporting muscle mass and overall health. Individuals with EPI may experience weight loss and muscle wasting due to malabsorption of nutrients and impaired digestion. Therefore, it's important for them to include adequate protein sources in their diet to maintain muscle mass and prevent further deterioration.

Good sources of protein include lean meats (such as chicken, turkey, and fish), eggs, dairy products (such as yogurt and cheese), tofu, legumes (such as beans and lentils), nuts, and seeds. When choosing protein sources, opt for lean options to minimize fat intake and reduce the risk of digestive discomfort associated with high-fat foods.

Fats:

Fats are another essential macronutrient that plays a crucial role in the body. They are a concentrated source of energy and provide essential fatty acids that the body cannot produce on its own. Fats are also involved in hormone production, cell membrane structure, and nutrient absorption.

In the context of EPI, dietary fats can pose challenges due to their potential to exacerbate digestive symptoms such as bloating, abdominal pain, and diarrhoea. However, not all fats are created equal, and choosing the right types of fats is key to supporting digestive health and overall well-being.

Healthy fats, such as monounsaturated and polyunsaturated fats, are beneficial for individuals with EPI as they are easier to digest compared to saturated and trans fats. Sources of healthy fats include avocados, nuts, seeds, olive oil, fatty fish (such as salmon and mackerel), and flaxseeds.

Carbohydrates:

Carbohydrates are the body's primary source of energy and play a crucial role in fuelling cellular processes, supporting brain function, and maintaining blood sugar levels. Carbohydrates are classified into simple carbohydrates (sugars) and complex carbohydrates (starches and fibres), each with varying effects on blood sugar levels and overall health.

In the context of managing EPI, carbohydrates can be an important source of energy and nutrients for individuals experiencing weight loss and malnutrition. However, it's important to choose carbohydrates wisely and prioritize complex carbohydrates that provide sustained energy and promote digestive health.

Good sources of complex carbohydrates include whole grains (such as brown rice, quinoa, oats, and barley), fruits, vegetables, legumes (such as beans and lentils), and starchy vegetables (such as sweet potatoes and squash). These foods are rich in fiber, vitamins, and minerals, and they are digested more slowly, helping to stabilize blood sugar levels and prevent energy crashes.

Simple carbohydrates, on the other hand, should be consumed in moderation, as they can cause rapid spikes and dips in blood sugar levels, leading to fluctuations in energy and mood. Limit intake of refined sugars, sugary snacks, desserts, and processed foods, and focus on whole, unprocessed carbohydrates for optimal health and well-being.

Vitamins and Minerals

Vitamins and minerals are micronutrients that are essential for various physiological functions in the body, including metabolism, immune function, and cellular health. While they are required in smaller quantities compared to macronutrients, vitamins and minerals play critical roles in supporting overall health and well-being. Let's explore the importance of vitamins and minerals in the diet and their relevance to managing Exocrine Pancreatic Insufficiency (EPI):

Vitamins:

Vitamins are organic compounds that are essential for various biochemical processes in the body. They are classified into two categories: fat-soluble vitamins (A, D, E, and K) and water-soluble vitamins (B vitamins and vitamin C). Each vitamin plays a unique role in supporting health and well-being, and deficiencies can lead to a range of health problems.

In the context of managing EPI, fat-soluble vitamins are of particular importance due to the impaired absorption of fats and fat-soluble nutrients associated with the condition. Individuals with EPI may be at risk of deficiencies in fat-soluble vitamins, leading to symptoms such as vision problems, bone disorders, and impaired immune function.

Good food sources of fat-soluble vitamins include:

- **Vitamin A:** Found in foods such as liver, carrots, sweet potatoes, spinach, and kale.

- **Vitamin D:** Found in fatty fish (such as salmon and mackerel), egg yolks, fortified dairy products, and sunlight exposure.

- **Vitamin E:** Found in nuts, seeds, vegetable oils, and leafy green vegetables.

- **Vitamin K:** Found in leafy green vegetables, broccoli, Brussels sprouts, and fermented foods (such as sauerkraut and kimchi).

Water-soluble vitamins, such as B vitamins and vitamin C, are also important for individuals with EPI as they play key roles in energy metabolism, nerve function, and immune health.

Good food sources of water-soluble vitamins include:

- **B vitamins:** Found in whole grains, lean meats, fish, poultry, eggs, dairy products, legumes, and leafy green vegetables.

- **Vitamin C:** Found in citrus fruits, strawberries, kiwi, bell peppers, broccoli, and tomatoes.

Minerals:

Minerals are inorganic compounds that are essential for various physiological processes in the body, including bone health, muscle function, and fluid balance. They are classified into two categories:

macro-minerals (required in larger quantities) and trace minerals (required in smaller quantities). Each mineral plays a unique role in supporting health and well-being, and deficiencies can lead to a range of health problems.

In the context of managing EPI, certain minerals are of particular importance due to their roles in supporting digestive health, bone health, and overall well-being. Individuals with EPI may be at risk of deficiencies in minerals such as calcium, magnesium, iron, and zinc, leading to symptoms such as osteoporosis, muscle weakness, anaemia, and impaired immune function.

Good food sources of these minerals include:

- Calcium: Found in dairy products (such as milk, yogurt, and cheese), leafy green vegetables, tofu, almonds, and fortified foods (such as fortified plant-based milk and orange juice).

- Magnesium: Found in nuts, seeds, whole grains, leafy green vegetables, legumes, and fortified foods (such as fortified breakfast cereals).

- Iron: Found in red meat, poultry, fish, tofu, lentils, beans, fortified cereals, and dark leafy green vegetables.

- Zinc: Found in meat, shellfish, poultry, nuts, seeds, legumes, whole grains, and dairy products.

CHAPTER FOUR

STOCKING YOUR PANTRY

EPI-Friendly Staples

In managing Exocrine Pancreatic Insufficiency (EPI), building a pantry stocked with EPI-friendly staples is essential for maintaining a nutritious diet while minimizing digestive discomfort. These staples provide the foundation for creating nourishing meals that are easy to digest and packed with essential nutrients.

Let's explore some key EPI-friendly staples and their role in supporting digestive health and overall well-being:

1. **Whole Grains:** Whole grains are a rich source of complex carbohydrates, fibre, vitamins, and minerals, making them an excellent choice for individuals with EPI. Opt for whole grain options such as brown rice, quinoa, oats, barley, and whole wheat pasta. These grains provide sustained energy, promote digestive health, and help stabilize blood sugar levels.

2. **Lean Proteins:** Incorporating lean sources of protein into your diet is essential for supporting muscle health and overall well-being. Choose lean proteins such as skinless poultry, fish, tofu, tempeh, legumes, and low-fat dairy products. These protein sources are easier to digest

compared to fatty cuts of meat and provide essential amino acids for muscle repair and growth.

3. **Healthy Fats:** Including healthy fats in moderation can help support digestive health and provide essential fatty acids that the body needs. Opt for sources of healthy fats such as avocados, nuts, seeds, olive oil, and fatty fish like salmon and mackerel. These fats are rich in monounsaturated and polyunsaturated fats, which can help reduce inflammation and support heart health.

4. **Fresh Fruits and Vegetables:** Fruits and vegetables are packed with vitamins, minerals, antioxidants, and fibre, making them essential components of an EPI-friendly diet. Choose a variety of colourful fruits and vegetables to ensure a diverse range of nutrients. Aim to incorporate a rainbow of colours into your meals, including leafy greens, berries, citrus fruits, cruciferous vegetables, and root vegetables.

5. **Low-Lactose Dairy Alternatives:** For individuals with lactose intolerance or difficulty digesting dairy products, opting for low-lactose or lactose-free dairy alternatives can be beneficial. Look for options such as lactose-free milk, yogurt, cheese, and plant-based milk alternatives like almond milk, soy milk, and oat milk. These alternatives provide calcium, vitamin D, and other essential nutrients without causing digestive discomfort.

6. **Herbs and Spices:** Adding herbs and spices to your meals can enhance flavor without adding extra fat or calories. Experiment with a variety of herbs and spices to add depth and complexity to your dishes. Common options include basil, cilantro, parsley, rosemary, thyme, garlic, ginger, turmeric, cumin, and paprika. These flavourful additions can help stimulate digestion and make meals more enjoyable.

7. **Enzyme Replacement Therapy (ERT):** While not a traditional pantry staple, enzyme replacement therapy (ERT) is a crucial component of managing EPI. ERT involves taking supplemental pancreatic enzymes with meals to aid in the digestion of food. These enzymes help compensate for the insufficient production of pancreatic enzymes, allowing for better nutrient absorption and reduced digestive symptoms.

Reading Labels for Hidden Ingredients

When managing Exocrine Pancreatic Insufficiency (EPI), reading labels for hidden ingredients is essential for avoiding foods that may exacerbate digestive symptoms and selecting products that are safe and suitable for your dietary needs. Many packaged and processed foods contain hidden ingredients that can be challenging to identify without careful scrutiny.

Let's explore some key tips for reading labels and navigating the grocery store with EPI:

1. **Check the Ingredient List:** Start by checking the ingredient list on packaged foods to identify any potential triggers or problematic ingredients. Look for common culprits such as high-fat ingredients, added sugars, artificial sweeteners, preservatives, and additives that may be difficult to digest or contribute to digestive discomfort.

2. **Look for High-Fat Ingredients:** Pay close attention to the types and amounts of fats used in packaged foods, as high-fat ingredients can exacerbate symptoms of EPI. Avoid products that contain excessive amounts of saturated and trans fats, which are often found in fried foods, baked goods, processed meats, and creamy sauces. Opt for products made with healthier fats such as monounsaturated and polyunsaturated fats, which are easier to digest and support heart health.

3. **Check for Added Sugars and Sweeteners:** Be mindful of added sugars and artificial sweeteners hidden in packaged foods, as they can contribute to spikes in blood sugar levels and exacerbate digestive symptoms. Look for ingredients such as cane sugar, high-fructose corn syrup, sucralose, aspartame, and saccharin on the label. Choose products with minimal added sugars and opt for natural sweeteners such as honey, maple syrup, and stevia when possible.

4. **Avoid Hidden Dairy Products:** If you have lactose intolerance or difficulty digesting dairy products, be vigilant about avoiding hidden sources of dairy in packaged foods. Look for ingredients such as milk, cheese, butter, cream, whey, and casein on the label. Opt for dairy-free alternatives or products labelled as lactose-free to minimize digestive discomfort.

5. **Check for Hidden Gluten:** If you have gluten intolerance or celiac disease, be on the lookout for hidden sources of gluten in packaged foods. Gluten can hide in ingredients such as wheat, barley, rye, malt, and modified food starch. Look for gluten-free certification labels or products labelled as gluten-free to ensure they are safe for consumption.

6. **Read Labels for Fiber Content:** While fibre is essential for digestive health, consuming excessive amounts of fibre-rich foods can exacerbate symptoms of EPI such as bloating and gas. Check the fibre content on packaged foods and choose products with moderate fibre content that won't overwhelm your digestive system. Opt for whole grains, fruits, and vegetables with soluble fibre, which is easier to digest than insoluble fibre.

7. **Be Mindful of Portion Sizes:** Pay attention to portion sizes listed on packaged foods and avoid consuming oversized servings, as this can overload your digestive system and lead to discomfort. Stick to recommended serving sizes and

listen to your body's hunger and fullness cues to prevent overeating.

CHAPTER FIVE

ESSENTIAL KITCHEN TOOLS FOR EPI DIET COOKING

Blender, Food Processor, and Others

In the realm of meal preparation and cooking, having the right tools can make all the difference. Blenders, food processors, and other kitchen appliances can streamline the cooking process, save time, and help individuals with Exocrine Pancreatic Insufficiency (EPI) create delicious and nutritious meals with ease. Let's delve into the roles and benefits of these kitchen appliances:

Blender:

Blenders are versatile kitchen appliances that are indispensable for individuals with EPI. They excel at blending and pureeing ingredients to create smoothies, soups, sauces, dips, and more. Blenders are particularly useful for individuals with EPI who may have difficulty digesting whole fruits and vegetables, as they can easily transform these ingredients into smooth, easily digestible liquids.

One of the primary benefits of using a blender for meal preparation is its ability to break down fibrous fruits and vegetables into a smooth consistency, making it easier for individuals with EPI to digest and absorb nutrients. Blending also helps retain the fiber content of fruits and vegetables, promoting digestive health and regularity.

Additionally, blenders are ideal for creating nutrient-dense smoothies and shakes that can serve as convenient meal replacements or snacks for individuals with EPI. By combining fruits, vegetables, protein sources, healthy fats, and other nutritious ingredients, individuals can create balanced and satisfying meals that support their nutritional needs.

Food Processor:

Food processors are another essential kitchen appliance for individuals with EPI, offering versatility and convenience for a wide range of food preparation tasks. Food processors excel at chopping, slicing, shredding, and pureeing ingredients, making them ideal for preparing ingredients for soups, salads, sauces, and dips.

One of the key benefits of using a food processor is its ability to quickly and efficiently chop and puree ingredients, saving time and effort in the kitchen. Food processors are particularly useful for individuals with EPI who may have difficulty chopping or handling certain foods due to digestive symptoms or physical limitations.

Food processors are also excellent for preparing large batches of food in advance, allowing individuals to stockpile pre-prepared ingredients for quick and easy meal assembly throughout the week. By chopping and prepping ingredients in bulk, individuals can streamline the cooking process and minimize time spent in the kitchen.

Other Kitchen Appliances:

In addition to blenders and food processors, there are several other kitchen appliances that can be invaluable for individuals with EPI:

1. **Slow Cooker:** Slow cookers are ideal for preparing hearty and nutritious meals with minimal effort. Simply add ingredients to the slow cooker in the morning, set the temperature, and let it simmer all day for a delicious meal ready by dinnertime.

2. **Instant Pot:** Instant pots are versatile multi-cookers that combine the functions of a pressure cooker, slow cooker, rice cooker, and more. They are perfect for preparing a wide range of meals quickly and efficiently, making them ideal for busy individuals with EPI.

3. **Immersion Blender:** Immersion blenders are handheld blenders that allow you to blend ingredients directly in the pot or container. They are convenient for pureeing soups, sauces, and other liquids without the need to transfer them to a traditional blender.

4. **Food Scale:** A food scale is a handy tool for measuring ingredients accurately, especially when following recipes or portioning meals. This can be particularly useful for

individuals with EPI who need to monitor their nutrient intake carefully.

Tips for Meal Preparation

Meal preparation is key for individuals with Exocrine Pancreatic Insufficiency (EPI) to ensure they have access to nourishing and easy-to-digest meals throughout the week. Here are some tips for effective meal preparation:

1. **Plan Ahead:** Take some time each week to plan your meals and snacks. Consider your schedule, dietary preferences, and nutritional needs when planning your meals. Make a list of ingredients you'll need and go grocery shopping to stock up on essentials.

2. **Batch Cooking:** Consider batch cooking large quantities of staple foods such as grains, proteins, and vegetables to have on hand for quick and easy meals throughout the week. Cook up a big pot of quinoa, brown rice, or lentils, grill or bake chicken breasts or tofu, and roast a variety of vegetables to have at the ready.

3. **Prep Ingredients:** Spend some time prepping ingredients in advance to streamline the cooking process during the week. Wash and chop fruits and vegetables, portion out snacks and ingredients for smoothies, and marinate proteins for easy cooking later on.

4. **Use Kitchen Appliances:** Take advantage of kitchen appliances such as blenders, food processors, slow cookers, and instant pots to make meal preparation easier and more efficient. These appliances can help you chop, puree, cook, and assemble meals with minimal effort.

5. **Portion Control:** Consider portioning out meals and snacks in advance to help you stick to appropriate serving sizes and avoid overeating. Use containers or meal prep trays to portion out meals and snacks for easy grab-and-go access throughout the week.

6. **Label and Store:** Once you've prepared your meals and snacks, label them with the date and contents and store them in the refrigerator or freezer as needed. Use airtight containers or resealable bags to keep food fresh and prevent spoilage.

7. **Experiment and Adapt:** Don't be afraid to experiment with new recipes, ingredients, and cooking techniques to keep your meals interesting and enjoyable. Be open to adapting recipes to suit your dietary needs and preferences, and don't hesitate to seek inspiration from cookbooks, websites, and cooking blogs

CHAPTER SIX

COMPREHENSIVE LIST OF EPI-FRIENDLY FOODS

Proteins

Food Name	Portion Size	Calories	Protein (g)	Fat (g)	Carbohydrates (g)	Fiber (g)
Almond Milk	1 cup	39	1	3	2	1
Bison	3 oz	152	24	6	0	0
Bison Jerky	1 oz	70	12	1	4	0
Black Beans	1/2 cup	114	8	0	20	8
Casein Protein Powder	1 scoop	120	24	1	3	0
Cheddar Cheese	1 oz	113	7	9	1	0
Chicken Breast	3 oz	140	26	3	0	0

Chicken Thigh	3 oz	177	21	10	0	0
Chickpeas	1/2 cup	134	7	2	22	6
Cod	3 oz	89	20	1	0	0
Cottage Cheese	1/2 cup	110	15	2	6	0
Cottage Cheese (2%)	1/2 cup	104	12	2	5	0
Crab	3 oz	82	17	1	0	0
Duck	3 oz	171	24	8	0	0
Edamame	1/2 cup	95	8	4	6	4
Egg Whites	3 large	51	11	0	1	0
Eggs	2 large	144	12	10	1	0
Elk	3 oz	145	22	6	0	0
Feta Cheese	1 oz	74	4	6	1	0

Goat Cheese	1 oz	75	5	6	0	0
Greek Yogurt	1 cup	130	23	0	9	0
Greek Yogurt (plain)	1 cup	130	23	0	9	0
Hemp Protein Powder	1 scoop	120	24	1	3	0
Lamb	3 oz	248	23	17	0	0
Lean Beef	3 oz	184	25	8	0	0
Lentils	1/2 cup	115	9	0	20	8
Lobster	3 oz	83	17	1	0	0
Mozzarella Cheese	1 oz	72	7	4	1	0
Parmesan Cheese	1 oz	122	10	8	1	0

Pea Protein Powder	1 scoop	120	24	1	3	0
Pork Tenderloin	3 oz	122	22	3	0	0
Quinoa	1/2 cup	111	4	2	19	2
Salmon	3 oz	177	22	10	0	0
Shrimp	3 oz	84	18	1	0	0
Skim Milk	1 cup	83	8	0	12	0
Soy Milk	1 cup	131	8	4	8	0
Swiss Cheese	1 oz	111	8	9	1	0
Tempeh	3 oz	162	15	9	9	0
Tilapia	3 oz	94	21	2	0	0
Tofu	3 oz	70	8	4	2	1
Tuna	3 oz	99	22	1	0	0

Turkey Breast	3 oz	135	26	1	0	0
Turkey Thigh	3 oz	147	21	7	0	0
Venison	3 oz	143	22	5	0	0
Whey Protein Powder	1 scoop	120	24	1	3	0

Fruits

Food Name	Portion Size	Calories	Carbohydrates (g)	Fiber (g)	Sugar (g)	Vitamin C (mg)
Apple	1 medium	95	25	4	19	8
Apricot	1 medium	17	4	1	3	3
Avocado	1/2 medium	114	6	5	0	10
Banana	1 medium	105	27	3	14	10
Blackberries	1 cup	62	14	8	7	30

Blood Orange	1 medium	62	15	3	12	70
Blueberries	1 cup	84	21	4	15	24
Cantaloupe	1 cup	53	13	1	13	68
Cherries	1 cup	87	22	3	18	10
Coconut	1 cup	283	12	7	6	6
Cranberries	1 cup	46	12	4	4	16
Dragon Fruit	1 medium	60	13	9	9	9
Gooseberries	1 cup	66	15	6	8	41
Grapefruit	1/2 medium	52	13	2	8	38
Grapes	1 cup	104	27	1	23	4
Guava	1 medium	37	8	3	5	231
Honeydew	1 cup	64	16	1	16	30
Jackfruit	1 cup	155	40	3	25	22

Kiwano (Horned Melon)	1 medium	103	22	7	17	96
Kiwi	1 medium	42	10	2	6	64
Kumquat	1 cup	71	16	9	9	73
Lemon	1 medium	17	5	2	1	30
Lime	1 medium	20	7	2	1	19
Lychee	1 cup	125	32	2	29	136
Mango	1 cup	99	25	3	23	60
Mango (Dried)	1 cup	336	86	6	63	112
Mulberries	1 cup	60	14	2	10	14
Nectarine	1 medium	62	15	2	11	7
Orange	1 medium	62	15	3	12	70
Papaya	1 cup	55	14	3	11	88
Passion Fruit	1 medium	17	4	9	4	70
Peach	1 medium	58	14	2	13	7
Pear	1 medium	101	27	6	17	7

Persimmon	1 medium	118	31	6	21	66
Pineapple	1 cup	82	22	2	16	79
Plantains	1 medium	218	57	4	31	55
Plum	1 medium	30	8	1	7	7
Pomegranate	1 medium	105	26	7	16	28
Pomelo	1 cup	72	18	2	12	128
Raspberries	1 cup	64	15	8	5	32
Starfruit	1 medium	28	6	2	4	34
Strawberries	1 cup	49	11	3	7	89
Tamarillo	1 medium	35	8	2	5	26
Tangerine	1 medium	47	12	2	9	26
Ugli Fruit	1 medium	47	11	3	9	51
Watermelon	1 cup	46	11	1	9	12

Vegetables

Food Name	Port ion Size	Calo ries	Carbohy drates (g)	Fib er (g)	Sug ar (g)	Vita min A (IU)	Vita min C (mg)
Articho ke	1 medi um	60	14	7	1	474	6
Aspara gus	1 cup	27	5	3	2	1014	7
Beetro ot	1 cup	59	13	4	9	58	6
Bell Pepper (green)	1 cup	30	7	3	3	1198	120
Bell Pepper (red)	1 cup	46	9	3	6	3726	190
Bell Pepper (yellow)	1 cup	50	12	2	9	1017	306

Bok Choy	1 cup	9	1	1	0	65	45
Broccoli	1 cup	55	11	5	2	567	81
Brussels Sprouts	1 cup	38	8	3	2	644	48
Cabbage (green)	1 cup	22	5	2	2	68	28
Carrot	1 medium	25	6	2	3	10191	7
Cauliflower	1 cup	27	5	2	2	0	46
Celery	1 stalk	6	1	1	0	449	3
Corn	1 cup	177	41	5	9	416	10
Cucumber	1 cup	16	4	1	1	62	4
Eggplant	1 cup	20	5	3	3	1239	2

Fennel	1 cup	27	6	2	3	838	10
Garlic	1 clove	4	1	0	0	0	1
Green Beans	1 cup	31	7	3	4	691	12
Kale	1 cup	33	6	1	1	10668	80
Kohlrabi	1 cup	36	8	4	5	0	84
Leek	1 cup	54	13	2	3	1022	17
Mushroom	1 cup	21	3	1	1	0	2
Okra	1 cup	31	7	3	1	621	22
Onion	1 medium	44	10	2	5	43	9
Peas	1 cup	118	21	8	8	1112	58
Potato	1 medium	161	37	4	2	0	48

Pumpkin	1 cup	49	12	3	3	599	12
Pumpkin (canned)	1 cup	49	12	3	3	599	12
Radish	1 cup	19	4	2	2	0	18
Rutabaga	1 cup	50	12	4	7	93	23
Snow Peas	1 cup	26	5	2	3	245	60
Spinach	1 cup	7	1	1	0	2813	8
Sprouts (alfalfa)	1 cup	8	1	1	0	4	8
Sprouts (bean)	1 cup	31	6	3	1	59	35
Squash (butternut)	1 cup	82	22	7	4	22831	31

Squash (summer)	1 cup	17	4		1	2	392	17
Sweet Potato	1 medium	103	24		4	7	21909	4
Swiss Chard	1 cup	7	1		1	0	214	10
Tomato	1 medium	22	5		1	3	1025	15
Turnip	1 medium	34	8		2	5	0	29
Turnip Greens	1 cup	18	4		2	1	6374	23
Watercress	1 cup	4	1		0	0	1122	3
Zucchini	1 cup	21	4		1	3	406	21

Grains

Food Name	Portion Size	Calories	Carbohydrates (g)	Fiber (g)	Protein (g)	Fat (g)
Amaranth	1/2 cup	134	23	3	5	2
Amaranth Flour	1/4 cup	130	24	3	5	2
Barley	1/2 cup	97	21	3	2	0
Barley Flakes	1/2 cup	100	23	4	2	0
Barley Flour	1/4 cup	110	24	4	3	0
Brown Rice	1/2 cup	108	22	2	2	1
Brown Rice Noodles	1/2 cup	110	24	1	2	0
Buckwheat	1/2 cup	155	33	5	6	1
Buckwheat Flour	1/4 cup	120	24	3	4	1

Buckwheat Noodles	1/2 cup	97	20	1	3	0
Bulgur	1/2 cup	76	17	4	3	0
Cornmeal	1/2 cup	400	87	7	9	4
Couscous	1/2 cup	112	23	2	4	0
Einkorn	1/2 cup	200	40	4	9	1
Farro	1/2 cup	97	20	3	4	0
Farro Flour	1/4 cup	120	25	2	4	0
Fonio	1/2 cup	335	70	3	8	1
Freekeh	1/2 cup	170	35	4	8	1
Kamut	1/2 cup	210	40	7	7	1

Kaniwa	1/2 cup	320	56	6	16	5
Millet	1/2 cup	207	41	2	6	2
Millet Flakes	1/2 cup	160	35	2	4	1
Millet Flour	1/4 cup	130	24	2	3	2
Oat Flour	1/4 cup	120	20	3	4	2
Oats	1/2 cup	154	27	4	6	3
Quinoa	1/2 cup	111	20	2	4	2
Quinoa Flour	1/4 cup	120	22	2	4	2
Rye	1/2 cup	100	22	4	4	1
Rye Flakes	1/2 cup	120	24	4	3	1
Sorghum	1/2 cup	316	68	6	10	3

Sorghum Flakes	1/2 cup	160	36		3	3	1
Sorghum Flour	1/4 cup	120	28		3	3	1
Spelt	1/2 cup	126	25		4	6	1
Spelt Flour	1/4 cup	110	23		4	4	0
Spelt Pasta	1/2 cup	174	36		4	6	1
Teff	1/2 cup	255	50		6	10	2
Teff Flakes	1/2 cup	160	35		4	6	1
Teff Flour	1/4 cup	140	29		4	6	1
Triticale	1/2 cup	199	40		6	7	1
Wheat Berries	1/2 cup	151	32		6	6	1

Whole Grain Bread	1 slice	69	12	2	3	1
Whole Wheat Flour	1/4 cup	110	23	4	4	0
Whole Wheat Pasta	1/2 cup	99	21	3	4	0
Whole Wheat Tortilla	1 tortilla	100	18	3	4	1

Dairy Alternatives

Food Name	Portion Size	Calories	Carbohydrates (g)	Protein (g)	Fat (g)	Calcium (mg)	Vitamin D (IU)
Almond Milk	1 cup	30	1	1	3	451	100
Barley Milk	1 cup	45	1	1	5	451	100

Black Sesame Milk	1 cup	50	2	2	4	451	100
Brazil Nut Milk	1 cup	50	1	0	5	450	0
Buckwheat Milk	1 cup	70	1	8	4	300	100
Cashew Milk	1 cup	25	1	0	2	451	100
Chia Seed Milk	1 cup	80	2	3	7	300	100
Chufa Milk	1 cup	50	1	0	5	451	100
Coconut Milk	1 cup	45	1	0	5	450	0
Flax Milk	1 cup	25	2	1	2	300	100
Hazelnut Milk	1 cup	100	1	2	10	300	100

Hemp Milk	1 cup	70	1	3	5	300	100
Hempseed Milk	1 cup	70	1	3	5	300	100
Lupin Milk	1 cup	60	1	4	3	300	100
Macadamia Milk	1 cup	50	1	0	5	450	0
Oat Milk	1 cup	120	16	3	5	350	144
Pea Milk	1 cup	70	1	8	4	300	100
Pecan Milk	1 cup	25	1	0	2	300	100
Pili Nut Milk	1 cup	100	1	0	5	450	0
Pistachio Milk	1 cup	100	1	2	10	300	100
Potato Milk	1 cup	100	18	1	3	300	100

Quinoa Milk	1 cup	70	12	2	1	300	100
Rice Bran Milk	1 cup	100	18	1	3	300	100
Rice Milk	1 cup	120	22	1	2	300	100
Safflower Milk	1 cup	80	2	3	7	300	100
Sesame Milk	1 cup	50	2	2	4	451	100
Sorghum Milk	1 cup	70	12	2	1	300	100
Soy Milk	1 cup	80	4	7	4	300	119
Sunflower Milk	1 cup	80	2	3	7	300	100
Tiger Nut Milk	1 cup	100	1	2	10	300	100

Walnut Milk	1 cup	45	1		1	5	450	0
Watermelon Seed Milk	1 cup	60	1		4	3	300	100
White Bean Milk	1 cup	70	1		8	4	300	100

Understanding Ingredients to Avoid or Limit

Managing Exocrine Pancreatic Insufficiency (EPI) involves more than just adding certain foods to your diet. Equally important is understanding which ingredients may exacerbate symptoms or hinder digestion. While each person's tolerance may vary, there are several common ingredients that individuals with EPI may benefit from avoiding or limiting.

Let's delve into these ingredients and understand their potential impact on EPI management.

1. High-Fat Foods:

Foods high in fat can be challenging for individuals with EPI to digest, as the pancreas produces insufficient enzymes to break down fats properly. As a result, undigested fats may cause symptoms like diarrhoea, bloating, and abdominal discomfort. High-fat foods to avoid or limit include fried foods, fatty meats, creamy sauces, full-fat dairy products, and heavily processed snacks like chips and pastries.

2. High-Fiber Foods:

While fibre is generally considered beneficial for digestive health, excessive fibre intake can be problematic for individuals with EPI. Fiber adds bulk to stools, which can exacerbate diarrhoea and contribute to malabsorption issues. Foods high in insoluble fibre, such as bran, whole grains, and some raw vegetables, may need to be limited. However, it's essential to maintain a balance, as some soluble fibre sources, like oats and certain fruits, can be beneficial in moderation.

3. Sugary Foods:

Consuming excessive amounts of sugar can disrupt blood sugar levels and exacerbate digestive symptoms in individuals with EPI. Sugary foods and beverages, including sweets, sugary cereals, soft drinks, and desserts, should be limited or avoided. Instead, focus on naturally sweet options like fruits (in moderation) and opt for low-sugar or sugar-free alternatives when possible.

4. Lactose-Containing Dairy Products:

Many individuals with EPI also have lactose intolerance, which means they lack the enzyme lactase needed to digest lactose, the sugar found in dairy products. Consuming lactose-containing dairy products can lead to symptoms such as bloating, gas, and diarrhoea. While some individuals may tolerate small amounts of lactose, others may need to avoid dairy altogether or opt for lactose-free alternatives like lactose-free milk and cheese.

5. Artificial Sweeteners and Sugar Alcohols:

While artificial sweeteners and sugar alcohols are marketed as low-calorie alternatives to sugar, they can have a laxative effect and exacerbate digestive symptoms in some individuals, including those with EPI. Common artificial sweeteners and sugar alcohols to be cautious of include sorbitol, mannitol, xylitol, aspartame, and sucralose. Reading food labels carefully and monitoring your body's response can help determine if these ingredients are problematic for you.

6. Spicy and Acidic Foods:

Spicy foods and acidic ingredients like citrus fruits, tomatoes, and vinegar can irritate the digestive tract and trigger symptoms like heartburn, acid reflux, and abdominal discomfort in individuals with EPI. While tolerance levels vary, it may be beneficial to limit these foods, especially if they exacerbate symptoms. Experimenting with milder spices and alternative flavourings can help add variety to your meals without causing digestive distress.

7. Processed and Refined Foods:

Processed and refined foods are often high in unhealthy fats, sugar, salt, and artificial additives, all of which can negatively impact digestive health and overall well-being. These foods include packaged snacks, ready-to-eat meals, fast food, and sugary cereals. Opting for whole, minimally processed foods like fresh fruits and vegetables, lean proteins, whole grains, and healthy fats can support better digestion and nutrient absorption.

8. Alcohol and Caffeine:

Alcohol and caffeine can both disrupt digestive function and exacerbate symptoms in individuals with EPI. Alcohol can interfere with pancreatic function and worsen malabsorption issues, while caffeine can stimulate gastric acid secretion and contribute to gastrointestinal discomfort. Moderating or avoiding alcohol and caffeine-containing beverages like coffee, tea, and energy drinks may help alleviate symptoms and promote better digestive health.

9. Gluten-Containing Foods:

Some individuals with EPI may also have gluten intolerance or celiac disease, which can cause inflammation and damage to the small intestine. Gluten is a protein found in wheat, barley, rye, and related grains. If you suspect gluten sensitivity, consider avoiding gluten-containing foods and opting for gluten-free alternatives like quinoa, rice, corn, and gluten-free oats.

10. Food Additives and Preservatives:

Certain food additives and preservatives, such as sulphites, nitrates, and MSG (monosodium glutamate), can trigger adverse reactions in some individuals, including digestive symptoms like bloating, gas, and abdominal pain. Reading food labels carefully and choosing products with minimal additives and preservatives can help reduce the risk of adverse reactions.

BREAKFAST RECIPES

Spinach and Mushroom Omelette

Ingredients:

- 2 large eggs
- 1 cup fresh spinach, chopped
- 1/2 cup mushrooms, sliced
- 1/4 cup shredded mozzarella cheese
- Salt and pepper to taste
- 1 teaspoon olive oil

Prep Time: 10 mins

Cooking Time: 10 mins

Total Time: 20 mins

Servings: 1

Nutrition Facts (per serving):

- 218 Calories
- Fat 15g
- Saturated fat 5g
- Cholesterol 380mg
- Sodium 387mg
- Carbohydrate 4g

- Protein 17g

- Fiber 1g

Instructions:

1. Heat olive oil in a non-stick skillet over medium heat.

2. Add mushrooms and spinach to the skillet and sauté until tender, about 3-4 minutes.

3. In a bowl, beat the eggs and season with salt and pepper.

4. Pour the beaten eggs into the skillet, covering the vegetables evenly.

5. Sprinkle shredded mozzarella cheese over the omelette.

6. Cook until the eggs are set and the cheese is melted, about 3-4 minutes.

7. Carefully fold the omelette in half and transfer to a plate. Serve hot.

Quinoa Breakfast Bowl

Ingredients:

- 1/2 cup cooked quinoa

- 1/4 cup Greek yogurt

- 1/2 cup mixed berries (strawberries, blueberries, raspberries)

- 1 tablespoon honey or maple syrup

- 1 tablespoon chopped nuts (almonds, walnuts, or pecans)

Prep Time: 5 mins

Cooking Time: 15 mins (for cooking quinoa, if not pre-cooked)

Total Time: 20 mins

Servings: 1

Nutrition Facts (per serving):

- 280 Calories

- Fat 6g

- Saturated fat 1g

- Cholesterol 5mg

- Sodium 22mg

- Carbohydrate 49g

- Protein 10g

- Fiber 6g

Instructions:

1. In a bowl, layer cooked quinoa, Greek yogurt, and mixed berries.

2. Drizzle honey or maple syrup over the top.

3. Sprinkle chopped nuts for added crunch and flavor.

4. Serve immediately as a nutritious and satisfying breakfast option.

Avocado Toast with Poached Egg

Ingredients:

- 1 slice whole grain bread
- 1/2 ripe avocado, mashed
- 1 large egg
- Salt and pepper to taste
- Optional toppings: cherry tomatoes, microgreens, feta cheese

Prep Time: 5 mins

Cooking Time: 5 mins

Total Time: 10 mins

Servings: 1

Nutrition Facts (per serving):

- 265 Calories
- Fat 16g
- Saturated fat 3g
- Cholesterol 185mg
- Sodium 280mg
- Carbohydrate 21g
- Protein 11g

- Fiber 8g

Instructions:

1. Toast the slice of whole grain bread until golden brown.

2. Spread mashed avocado evenly on top of the toast.

3. Fill a small saucepan with water and bring to a simmer. Crack the egg into a small bowl.

4. Carefully slide the egg into the simmering water and poach for 3-4 minutes, until the egg whites are set but the yolk is still runny.

5. Use a slotted spoon to remove the poached egg from the water and place it on top of the avocado toast.

6. Season with salt and pepper to taste.

7. Garnish with optional toppings like cherry tomatoes, microgreens, or crumbled feta cheese if desired.

Banana and Peanut Butter Smoothie

Ingredients:

- 1 ripe banana, peeled and sliced

- 1 tablespoon natural peanut butter

- 1/2 cup Greek yogurt

- 1/2 cup unsweetened almond milk

- 1 tablespoon honey or maple syrup (optional)

- Ice cubes

Prep Time: 5 mins

Cooking Time: 0 mins

Total Time: 5 mins

Servings: 1

Nutrition Facts (per serving):

- 290 Calories

- Fat 10g

- Saturated fat 2g

- Cholesterol 5mg

- Sodium 220mg

- Carbohydrate 39g

- Protein 15g

- Fiber 5g

Instructions:

1. In a blender, combine sliced banana, peanut butter, Greek yogurt, almond milk, and honey or maple syrup if using.

2. Add a handful of ice cubes to the blender.

3. Blend on high speed until smooth and creamy.

4. Pour the smoothie into a glass and serve immediately as a refreshing and nutritious breakfast option.

Chia Seed Pudding with Berries

Ingredients:

- 2 tablespoons chia seeds

- 1/2 cup unsweetened almond milk

- 1/2 teaspoon vanilla extract

- 1 tablespoon honey or maple syrup

- 1/2 cup mixed berries (strawberries, blueberries, raspberries)

- Optional toppings: sliced almonds, shredded coconut

Prep Time: 5 mins (plus chilling time)

Cooking Time: 0 mins

Total Time: 5 mins (plus chilling time)

Servings: 1

Nutrition Facts (per serving):

- 200 Calories

- Fat 9g

- Saturated fat 1g

- Cholesterol 0mg

- Sodium 80mg

- Carbohydrate 28g

- Protein 5g

- Fiber 10g

Instructions:

1. In a bowl or jar, combine chia seeds, almond milk, vanilla extract, and honey or maple syrup.

2. Stir well to combine and ensure that the chia seeds are evenly distributed.

3. Cover and refrigerate for at least 2 hours or overnight, until the mixture thickens and forms a pudding-like consistency.

4. Before serving, top the chia seed pudding with mixed berries and optional toppings like sliced almonds or shredded coconut.

5. Enjoy chilled as a nutritious and satisfying breakfast or snack option.

Vegetable Frittata

Ingredients:

- 4 large eggs

- 1/4 cup milk or dairy-free alternative

- 1/2 cup diced bell peppers

- 1/2 cup diced tomatoes

- 1/2 cup chopped spinach

- 1/4 cup diced onions

- Salt and pepper to taste

- 1 tablespoon olive oil

Prep Time: 10 mins

Cooking Time: 15 mins

Total Time: 25 mins

Servings: 2

Nutrition Facts (per serving):

- 180 Calories

- Fat 12g

- Saturated fat 3g

- Cholesterol 190mg

- Sodium 210mg

- Carbohydrate 7g

- Protein 11g

- Fiber 2g

Instructions:

1. Preheat the oven to 350°F (175°C).

2. In a bowl, whisk together eggs, milk, salt, and pepper.

3. Heat olive oil in an oven-safe skillet over medium heat.

4. Add onions, bell peppers, and tomatoes to the skillet. Cook until softened, about 5 minutes.

5. Add spinach to the skillet and cook until wilted.

6. Pour the egg mixture over the vegetables in the skillet.

7. Cook on the stovetop for 2-3 minutes until the edges start to set.

8. Transfer the skillet to the preheated oven and bake for 10-12 minutes until the frittata is set and golden brown.

9. Slice and serve hot.

Apple Cinnamon Overnight Oats

Ingredients:

- 1/2 cup rolled oats

- 1/2 cup unsweetened almond milk

- 1/2 medium apple, diced

- 1 tablespoon maple syrup or honey

- 1/2 teaspoon ground cinnamon

- 1 tablespoon chopped walnuts or almonds

Prep Time: 5 mins (plus chilling time)

Cooking Time: 0 mins

Total Time: 5 mins (plus chilling time)

Servings: 1

Nutrition Facts (per serving):

- 250 Calories

- Fat 8g

- Saturated fat 1g

- Cholesterol 0mg

- Sodium 90mg

- Carbohydrate 42g

- Protein 5g

- Fiber 7g

Instructions:

1. In a mason jar or container, combine rolled oats, almond milk, diced apple, maple syrup or honey, and ground cinnamon.

2. Stir well to combine all ingredients.

3. Cover and refrigerate overnight or for at least 4 hours.

4. Before serving, stir the overnight oats and top with chopped nuts.

5. Enjoy cold as a convenient and nutritious breakfast option.

Sweet Potato Hash with Eggs

Ingredients:

- 1 medium sweet potato, peeled and diced

- 1/2 bell pepper, diced

- 1/4 cup diced onions

- 2 large eggs

- 1 tablespoon olive oil

- Salt and pepper to taste

- Optional toppings: avocado slices, hot sauce

Prep Time: 10 mins

Cooking Time: 15 mins

Total Time: 25 mins

Servings: 2

Nutrition Facts (per serving):

- 220 Calories

- Fat 13g

- Saturated fat 3g

- Cholesterol 190mg

- Sodium 120mg

- Carbohydrate 18g

- Protein 8g

- Fiber 3g

Instructions:

1. Heat olive oil in a skillet over medium heat.

2. Add diced sweet potato to the skillet and cook until slightly softened, about 5 minutes.

3. Add diced bell pepper and onions to the skillet. Cook until vegetables are tender, about 5 minutes.

4. Create wells in the sweet potato hash and crack an egg into each well.

5. Season eggs with salt and pepper.

6. Cover the skillet and cook until the eggs are cooked to your desired doneness, about 5 minutes for runny yolks.

7. Serve hot with optional toppings like avocado slices or hot sauce.

Greek Yogurt Parfait

Ingredients:

- 1/2 cup Greek yogurt

- 1/4 cup granola

- 1/4 cup mixed berries (strawberries, blueberries, raspberries)

- 1 tablespoon honey or maple syrup

Prep Time: 5 mins

Cooking Time: 0 mins

Total Time: 5 mins

Servings: 1

Nutrition Facts (per serving):

- 220 Calories

- Fat 6g

- Saturated fat 1g

- Cholesterol 5mg

- Sodium 80mg

- Carbohydrate 34g

- Protein 10g

- Fiber 4g

Instructions:

1. In a glass or bowl, layer Greek yogurt, granola, and mixed berries.

2. Drizzle honey or maple syrup over the top.

3. Repeat layers if desired.

4. Serve immediately as a delicious and nutritious breakfast or snack option.

Turkey and Veggie Breakfast Burrito

Ingredients:

- 2 large eggs, lightly beaten

- 2 slices turkey bacon, chopped

- 1/4 cup diced bell peppers

- 1/4 cup diced onions

- 2 tablespoons shredded cheddar cheese

- 2 whole wheat or gluten-free tortillas

- Salt and pepper to taste

- Olive oil for cooking

Prep Time: 10 mins

Cooking Time: 10 mins

Total Time: 20 mins

Servings: 2

Nutrition Facts (per serving):

- 270 Calories

- Fat 15g

- Saturated fat 5g

- Cholesterol 210mg

- Sodium 380mg

- Carbohydrate 20g

- Protein 16g

- Fiber 3g

Instructions:

1. Heat olive oil in a skillet over medium heat.

2. Add chopped turkey bacon to the skillet and cook until crispy, about 5 minutes.

3. Add diced bell peppers and onions to the skillet. Cook until vegetables are tender, about 3-4 minutes.

4. Pour beaten eggs over the turkey and vegetables in the skillet.

5. Season with salt and pepper to taste.

6. Cook, stirring occasionally, until the eggs are scrambled and cooked through.

7. Sprinkle shredded cheddar cheese over the egg mixture and stir until melted.

8. Warm tortillas in a separate skillet or microwave.

9. Divide the egg mixture evenly between the tortillas and roll into burritos.

10. Serve hot as a satisfying and protein-packed breakfast option.

LUNCH RECIPES

Quinoa and Black Bean Salad

Ingredients:

- 1 cup cooked quinoa

- 1/2 cup black beans, drained and rinsed

- 1/2 cup diced bell peppers (any color)

- 1/4 cup diced red onions

- 1/4 cup chopped fresh cilantro

- Juice of 1 lime

- 1 tablespoon olive oil

- Salt and pepper to taste

- Optional toppings: avocado slices, crumbled feta cheese

Prep Time: 10 mins (if quinoa is pre-cooked)

Cooking Time: 0 mins

Total Time: 10 mins

Servings: 2

Nutrition Facts (per serving):

- 250 Calories

- Fat 8g

- Saturated fat 1g

- Cholesterol 0mg

- Sodium 160mg

- Carbohydrate 38g

- Protein 9g

- Fiber 9g

Instructions:

1. In a large bowl, combine cooked quinoa, black beans, diced bell peppers, red onions, and chopped cilantro.

2. Drizzle olive oil and lime juice over the salad.

3. Season with salt and pepper to taste.

4. Toss well to combine all ingredients evenly.

5. Divide the salad into serving bowls.

6. Top with optional toppings like avocado slices or crumbled feta cheese if desired.

7. Serve chilled or at room temperature.

Turkey and Vegetable Stir-Fry

Ingredients:

- 8 ounces turkey breast, thinly sliced

- 2 cups mixed vegetables (broccoli, bell peppers, snap peas)

- 2 tablespoons low-sodium soy sauce

- 1 tablespoon olive oil

- 2 cloves garlic, minced

- 1 teaspoon grated ginger

- 1 tablespoon cornstarch

- Salt and pepper to taste

- Cooked brown rice or quinoa for serving

Prep Time: 15 mins

Cooking Time: 10 mins

Total Time: 25 mins

Servings: 2

Nutrition Facts (per serving, without rice/quinoa):

- 220 Calories

- Fat 8g

- Saturated fat 1g

- Cholesterol 50mg

- Sodium 350mg

- Carbohydrate 10g

- Protein 25g

- Fiber 3g

Instructions:

1. In a small bowl, whisk together soy sauce, garlic, ginger, and cornstarch. Set aside.

2. Heat olive oil in a large skillet or wok over medium-high heat.

3. Add sliced turkey breast to the skillet and stir-fry until cooked through, about 5-6 minutes.

4. Add mixed vegetables to the skillet and continue to stir-fry for another 3-4 minutes until vegetables are tender-crisp.

5. Pour the soy sauce mixture over the turkey and vegetables in the skillet.

6. Stir well to coat everything evenly and cook for an additional 1-2 minutes until the sauce thickens.

7. Season with salt and pepper to taste.

8. Serve hot over cooked brown rice or quinoa.

Salmon and Asparagus Foil Packets

Ingredients:

- 2 salmon fillets

- 1 bunch asparagus, trimmed

- 2 tablespoons olive oil

- 2 cloves garlic, minced

- 1 lemon, thinly sliced

- Salt and pepper to taste

- Fresh dill for garnish

Prep Time: 10 mins

Cooking Time: 20 mins

Total Time: 30 mins

Servings: 2

Nutrition Facts (per serving):

- 320 Calories

- Fat 20g

- Saturated fat 3g

- Cholesterol 80mg

- Sodium 200mg

- Carbohydrate 7g

- Protein 30g

- Fiber 4g

Instructions:

1. Preheat the oven to 400°F (200°C).

2. Cut two large pieces of aluminium foil.

3. Place a salmon fillet in the centre of each piece of foil.

4. Arrange asparagus spears around the salmon fillets.

5. Drizzle olive oil over the salmon and asparagus.

6. Sprinkle minced garlic over the salmon and asparagus.

7. Season with salt and pepper to taste.

8. Place lemon slices on top of the salmon.

9. Fold the edges of the foil to create a sealed packet.

10. Place the foil packets on a baking sheet and bake in the preheated oven for 15-20 minutes until the salmon is cooked through and the asparagus is tender.

11. Carefully open the foil packets and transfer the contents to serving plates.

12. Garnish with fresh dill and serve hot.

Mediterranean Chickpea Salad

Ingredients:

- 1 can (15 ounces) chickpeas, drained and rinsed

- 1 cup cherry tomatoes, halved

- 1/2 cucumber, diced

- 1/4 cup diced red onion

- 1/4 cup chopped fresh parsley

- 1/4 cup crumbled feta cheese

- 2 tablespoons olive oil

- 1 tablespoon red wine vinegar

- Salt and pepper to taste

Prep Time: 10 mins

Cooking Time: 0 mins

Total Time: 10 mins

Servings: 2

Nutrition Facts (per serving):

- 290 Calories

- Fat 14g

- Saturated fat 3g

- Cholesterol 8mg

- Sodium 280mg

- Carbohydrate 34g

- Protein 10g

- Fiber 9g

Instructions:

1. In a large bowl, combine chickpeas, cherry tomatoes, cucumber, red onion, parsley, and feta cheese.

2. Drizzle olive oil and red wine vinegar over the salad.

3. Season with salt and pepper to taste.

4. Toss well to coat all ingredients evenly.

5. Serve chilled as a refreshing and nutritious lunch option.

Vegetable and Tofu Stir-Fry

Ingredients:

- 8 ounces firm tofu, drained and cubed

- 2 cups mixed vegetables (bell peppers, broccoli, carrots)

- 2 tablespoons low-sodium soy sauce

- 1 tablespoon sesame oil

- 2 cloves garlic, minced

- 1 teaspoon grated ginger

- 1 tablespoon cornstarch

- Cooked brown rice or quinoa for serving

Prep Time: 15 mins

Cooking Time: 10 mins

Total Time: 25 mins

Servings: 2

Nutrition Facts (per serving, without rice/quinoa):

- 180 Calories

- Fat 8g

- Saturated fat 1g

- Cholesterol 0mg

- Sodium 350mg

- Carbohydrate 14g

- Protein 12g

- Fiber 4g

Instructions:

1. In a small bowl, whisk together soy sauce, sesame oil, garlic, ginger, and cornstarch. Set aside.

2. Heat olive oil in a large skillet or wok over medium-high heat.

3. Add cubed tofu to the skillet and stir-fry until golden brown, about 5-6 minutes.

4. Add mixed vegetables to the skillet and continue to stir-fry for another 3-4 minutes until vegetables are tender-crisp.

5. Pour the soy sauce mixture over the tofu and vegetables in the skillet.

6. Stir well to coat everything evenly and cook for an additional 1-2 minutes until the sauce thickens.

7. Serve hot over cooked brown rice or quinoa.

Turkey and Quinoa Stuffed Bell Peppers

Ingredients:

- 4 large bell peppers (any color)
- 1 cup cooked quinoa
- 1/2 pound ground turkey
- 1/2 cup diced tomatoes
- 1/4 cup diced onions
- 1/4 cup shredded mozzarella cheese
- 1 teaspoon olive oil
- Salt and pepper to taste
- Optional toppings: chopped fresh parsley, hot sauce

Prep Time: 15 mins

Cooking Time: 30 mins

Total Time: 45 mins

Servings: 4

Nutrition Facts (per serving):

- 250 Calories
- Fat 9g
- Saturated fat 3g
- Cholesterol 40mg

- Sodium 180mg

- Carbohydrate 20g

- Protein 20g

- Fiber 4g

Instructions:

1. Preheat the oven to 375°F (190°C).

2. Cut the tops off the bell peppers and remove the seeds and membranes.

3. In a skillet, heat olive oil over medium heat.

4. Add ground turkey and diced onions to the skillet. Cook until turkey is browned and onions are softened, about 5-7 minutes.

5. Stir in cooked quinoa and diced tomatoes. Season with salt and pepper to taste.

6. Stuff the bell peppers with the turkey-quinoa mixture and place them in a baking dish.

7. Sprinkle shredded mozzarella cheese over the stuffed peppers.

8. Cover the baking dish with foil and bake in the preheated oven for 25-30 minutes until the peppers are tender.

9. Remove foil and bake for an additional 5 minutes until the cheese is melted and bubbly.

10. Garnish with chopped fresh parsley and serve hot with optional toppings like hot sauce.

Chickpea and Spinach Salad with Lemon-Tahini Dressing

Ingredients:

- 1 can (15 ounces) chickpeas, drained and rinsed

- 2 cups fresh baby spinach

- 1/4 cup diced red onions

- 1/4 cup diced cucumbers

- 1/4 cup diced tomatoes

- 2 tablespoons chopped fresh parsley

- 2 tablespoons tahini

- Juice of 1 lemon

- 1 tablespoon olive oil

- Salt and pepper to taste

Prep Time: 10 mins

Cooking Time: 0 mins

Total Time: 10 mins

Servings: 2

Nutrition Facts (per serving):

- 280 Calories

- Fat 14g

- Saturated fat 2g

- Cholesterol 0mg

- Sodium 280mg

- Carbohydrate 32g

- Protein 10g

- Fiber 8g

Instructions:

1. In a large bowl, combine chickpeas, baby spinach, diced red onions, cucumbers, tomatoes, and chopped parsley.

2. In a small bowl, whisk together tahini, lemon juice, olive oil, salt, and pepper to make the dressing.

3. Pour the dressing over the salad and toss well to coat all ingredients evenly.

4. Serve immediately as a refreshing and nutritious lunch option.

Vegetable and Lentil Soup

Ingredients:

- 1 cup dried green or brown lentils, rinsed

- 4 cups vegetable broth

- 1 cup diced carrots

- 1 cup diced celery

- 1 cup diced onions

- 2 cloves garlic, minced

- 1 teaspoon dried thyme

- 1 teaspoon dried oregano

- Salt and pepper to taste

- 2 tablespoons olive oil

Prep Time: 10 mins

Cooking Time: 30 mins

Total Time: 40 mins

Servings: 4

Nutrition Facts (per serving):

- 220 Calories

- Fat 6g

- Saturated fat 1g

- Cholesterol 0mg

- Sodium 480mg

- Carbohydrate 32g

- Protein 12g

- Fiber 12g

Instructions:

1. In a large pot, heat olive oil over medium heat.

2. Add diced onions, carrots, and celery to the pot. Cook until vegetables are softened, about 5-7 minutes.

3. Add minced garlic, dried thyme, and dried oregano to the pot. Cook for an additional 1-2 minutes until fragrant.

4. Pour vegetable broth into the pot and bring to a simmer.

5. Add rinsed lentils to the pot and stir well to combine.

6. Cover the pot and simmer for 20-25 minutes until lentils are tender.

7. Season with salt and pepper to taste.

8. Serve hot as a comforting and nutritious lunch option.

Tuna Salad Lettuce Wraps

Ingredients:

- 2 cans (5 ounces each) tuna, drained

- 1/4 cup diced celery

- 1/4 cup diced red onions

- 2 tablespoons mayonnaise or Greek yogurt

- 1 tablespoon Dijon mustard

- 1 tablespoon lemon juice

- Salt and pepper to taste

- 4 large lettuce leaves (romaine or iceberg)

- Optional toppings: sliced avocado, cherry tomatoes

Prep Time: 10 mins

Cooking Time: 0 mins

Total Time: 10 mins

Servings: 2

Nutrition Facts (per serving):

- 220 Calories

- Fat 10g

- Saturated fat 1g

- Cholesterol 40mg

- Sodium 360mg

- Carbohydrate 5g

- Protein 25g

- Fiber 2g

Instructions:

1. In a bowl, combine drained tuna, diced celery, diced red onions, mayonnaise or Greek yogurt, Dijon mustard, and lemon juice.

2. Mix well to combine all ingredients evenly.

3. Season with salt and pepper to taste.

4. Spoon tuna salad mixture onto lettuce leaves.

5. Top with optional toppings like sliced avocado or cherry tomatoes if desired.

6. Roll up the lettuce leaves to form wraps.

7. Serve immediately as a light and protein-packed lunch option.

Chicken and Vegetable Skewers

Ingredients:

- 1 pound boneless, skinless chicken breast, cut into cubes

- 2 cups mixed vegetables (bell peppers, zucchini, cherry tomatoes)

- 2 tablespoons olive oil

- 2 cloves garlic, minced

- 1 teaspoon dried oregano

- Salt and pepper to taste

- Wooden or metal skewers

Prep Time: 15 mins

Cooking Time: 15 mins

Total Time: 30 mins

Servings: 4

Nutrition Facts (per serving):

- 280 Calories

- Fat 10g

- Saturated fat 2g

- Cholesterol 80mg

- Sodium 180mg

- Carbohydrate 10g

- Protein 35g

- Fiber 3g

Instructions:

1. If using wooden skewers, soak them in water for 30 minutes to prevent burning.

2. In a bowl, combine olive oil, minced garlic, dried oregano, salt, and pepper.

3. Thread chicken cubes and mixed vegetables onto skewers, alternating as desired.

4. Brush olive oil mixture over the skewers.

5. Preheat a grill or grill pan over medium-high heat.

6. Grill the skewers for 10-12 minutes, turning occasionally, until the chicken is cooked through and the vegetables are tender.

7. Serve hot with optional sides like rice or quinoa.

DINNER RECIPES

Grilled Lemon Herb Chicken

Ingredients:

- 4 boneless, skinless chicken breasts
- 2 tablespoons olive oil
- 2 cloves garlic, minced
- Zest and juice of 1 lemon
- 1 tablespoon chopped fresh parsley
- 1 tablespoon chopped fresh thyme
- Salt and pepper to taste

Prep Time: 10 mins

Marinating Time: 30 mins

Cooking Time: 15 mins

Total Time: 55 mins

Servings: 4

Nutrition Facts (per serving):

- 220 Calories
- Fat 10g
- Saturated fat 2g
- Cholesterol 80mg

- Sodium 180mg

- Carbohydrate 0g

- Protein 30g

Instructions:

1. In a bowl, whisk together olive oil, minced garlic, lemon zest, lemon juice, chopped parsley, chopped thyme, salt, and pepper.

2. Place chicken breasts in a shallow dish and pour the marinade over them. Cover and refrigerate for at least 30 minutes.

3. Preheat grill to medium-high heat.

4. Remove chicken from marinade and discard excess marinade.

5. Grill chicken breasts for 6-8 minutes per side, or until internal temperature reaches 165°F (74°C) and juices run clear.

6. Remove from grill and let rest for 5 minutes before serving.

7. Serve hot with your choice of side dishes, such as roasted vegetables or quinoa.

Baked Salmon with Garlic-Herb Butter

Ingredients:

- 4 salmon fillets

- 4 tablespoons unsalted butter, softened

- 2 cloves garlic, minced

- 1 tablespoon chopped fresh parsley

- 1 tablespoon chopped fresh dill

- 1 tablespoon lemon juice

- Salt and pepper to taste

Prep Time: 10 mins

Cooking Time: 15 mins

Total Time: 25 mins

Servings: 4

Nutrition Facts (per serving):

- 280 Calories

- Fat 18g

- Saturated fat 7g

- Cholesterol 90mg

- Sodium 150mg

- Carbohydrate 1g

- Protein 28g

Instructions:

1. Preheat oven to 375°F (190°C).

2. In a small bowl, combine softened butter, minced garlic, chopped parsley, chopped dill, lemon juice, salt, and pepper.

3. Place salmon fillets on a baking sheet lined with parchment paper.

4. Spread garlic-herb butter evenly over the tops of the salmon fillets.

5. Bake in the preheated oven for 12-15 minutes, or until salmon flakes easily with a fork and reaches an internal temperature of 145°F (63°C).

6. Remove from oven and let rest for a few minutes before serving.

7. Serve hot with steamed vegetables or a mixed green salad.

Vegetarian Chickpea Curry

Ingredients:

- 2 tablespoons olive oil

- 1 onion, finely chopped

- 2 cloves garlic, minced

- 1 tablespoon grated fresh ginger

- 2 teaspoons curry powder

- 1 teaspoon ground cumin

- 1 teaspoon ground turmeric

- 1 can (15 ounces) chickpeas, drained and rinsed

- 1 can (14 ounces) diced tomatoes

- 1 can (14 ounces) coconut milk

- Salt and pepper to taste

- Fresh cilantro for garnish

Prep Time: 10 mins

Cooking Time: 20 mins

Total Time: 30 mins

Servings: 4

Nutrition Facts (per serving):

- 320 Calories

- Fat 20g

- Saturated fat 10g

- Cholesterol 0mg

- Sodium 280mg

- Carbohydrate 30g

- Protein 8g

Instructions:

1. Heat olive oil in a large skillet over medium heat.

2. Add chopped onion to the skillet and cook until softened, about 3-4 minutes.

3. Add minced garlic, grated ginger, curry powder, ground cumin, and ground turmeric to the skillet. Cook for an additional 1-2 minutes until fragrant.

4. Stir in drained chickpeas, diced tomatoes, and coconut milk.

5. Season with salt and pepper to taste.

6. Simmer the curry for 15-20 minutes, stirring occasionally, until thickened.

7. Serve hot, garnished with fresh cilantro, over cooked rice or quinoa.

Beef and Broccoli Stir-Fry

Ingredients:

- 1 pound flank steak, thinly sliced

- 1/4 cup low-sodium soy sauce

- 2 tablespoons oyster sauce

- 1 tablespoon brown sugar

- 2 cloves garlic, minced

- 1 teaspoon grated fresh ginger

- 2 tablespoons olive oil

- 2 cups broccoli florets

- Cooked brown rice for serving

Prep Time: 15 mins

Cooking Time: 15 mins

Total Time: 30 mins

Servings: 4

Nutrition Facts (per serving):

- 320 Calories

- Fat 15g

- Saturated fat 4g

- Cholesterol 80mg

- Sodium 580mg

- Carbohydrate 12g

- Protein 35g

Instructions:

1. In a bowl, whisk together soy sauce, oyster sauce, brown sugar, minced garlic, and grated ginger.

2. Place thinly sliced flank steak in a shallow dish and pour half of the sauce over it. Toss to coat evenly and let marinate for 10-15 minutes.

3. Heat olive oil in a large skillet or wok over high heat.

4. Add marinated beef to the skillet and stir-fry for 2-3 minutes until browned.

5. Remove beef from skillet and set aside.

6. In the same skillet, add broccoli florets and stir-fry for 3-4 minutes until tender-crisp.

7. Return beef to the skillet and pour in the remaining sauce.

8. Stir well to coat everything evenly and cook for an additional 1-2 minutes.

9. Serve hot over cooked brown rice.

Vegetable and Tofu Stir-Fry

Ingredients:

- 1 block (14 ounces) firm tofu, drained and cubed

- 2 tablespoons low-sodium soy sauce

- 1 tablespoon sesame oil

- 2 cloves garlic, minced

- 1 teaspoon grated fresh ginger

- 1 tablespoon cornstarch

- 2 tablespoons olive oil

- 2 cups mixed vegetables (bell peppers, broccoli, carrots)

- Cooked brown rice for serving

Prep Time: 15 mins

Cooking Time: 15 mins

Total Time: 30 mins

Servings: 4

Nutrition Facts (per serving, without rice):

- 280 Calories

- Fat 15g

- Saturated fat 2g

- Cholesterol 0mg

- Sodium 350mg

- Carbohydrate 20g

- Protein 15g

Instructions:

1. In a small bowl, whisk together soy sauce, sesame oil, minced garlic, grated ginger, and cornstarch. Set aside.

2. Heat olive oil in a large skillet or wok over medium-high heat.

3. Add cubed tofu to the skillet and stir-fry until golden brown, about 5-6 minutes.

4. Remove tofu from skillet and set aside.

5. In the same skillet, add mixed vegetables and stir-fry for 3-4 minutes until tender-crisp.

6. Return tofu to the skillet and pour the soy sauce mixture over the tofu and vegetables.

7. Stir well to coat everything evenly and cook for an additional 1-2 minutes until the sauce thickens.

8. Serve hot over cooked brown rice.

Quinoa Stuffed Bell Peppers

Ingredients:

- 4 large bell peppers (any colour)

- 1 cup cooked quinoa

- 1/2 cup black beans, drained and rinsed

- 1/2 cup corn kernels (fresh or frozen)

- 1/2 cup diced tomatoes

- 1/4 cup diced onions

- 1/4 cup diced green chilies

- 1 teaspoon ground cumin

- 1/2 teaspoon chili powder

- Salt and pepper to taste

- 1/4 cup shredded cheddar cheese (optional)

- Fresh cilantro for garnish

Prep Time: 15 mins

Cooking Time: 30 mins

Total Time: 45 mins

Servings: 4

Nutrition Facts (per serving):

- 250 Calories

- Fat 5g

- Saturated fat 2g

- Cholesterol 10mg

- Sodium 280mg

- Carbohydrate 45g

- Protein 9g

- Fiber 9g

Instructions:

1. Preheat the oven to 375°F (190°C). Cut the tops off the bell peppers and remove the seeds and membranes.

2. In a large bowl, combine cooked quinoa, black beans, corn kernels, diced tomatoes, diced onions, diced green chilies, ground cumin, chili powder, salt, and pepper. Mix well.

3. Stuff the bell peppers with the quinoa mixture and place them in a baking dish.

4. If desired, sprinkle shredded cheddar cheese on top of the stuffed peppers.

5. Cover the baking dish with foil and bake in the preheated oven for 25-30 minutes until the peppers are tender.

6. Remove foil and bake for an additional 5 minutes until the cheese is melted and bubbly.

7. Garnish with fresh cilantro before serving.

Mushroom and Spinach Risotto

Ingredients:

- 1 tablespoon olive oil

- 1 small onion, finely chopped

- 2 cloves garlic, minced

- 1 cup Arborio rice

- 1/2 cup dry white wine (optional)

- 4 cups vegetable broth, heated

- 8 ounces mushrooms, sliced

- 2 cups baby spinach leaves

- 1/4 cup grated Parmesan cheese

- Salt and pepper to taste

- Fresh parsley for garnish

Prep Time: 10 mins

Cooking Time: 30 mins

Total Time: 40 mins

Servings: 4

Nutrition Facts (per serving):

- 300 Calories

- Fat 6g

- Saturated fat 2g

- Cholesterol 5mg

- Sodium 720mg

- Carbohydrate 45g

- Protein 8g

- Fiber 3g

Instructions:

1. Heat olive oil in a large skillet over medium heat. Add chopped onion and minced garlic, and cook until softened, about 3-4 minutes.

2. Add Arborio rice to the skillet and cook for 1-2 minutes until translucent.

3. If using, pour in the white wine and cook until evaporated, stirring constantly.

4. Begin adding the heated vegetable broth to the skillet, one ladleful at a time, stirring constantly until absorbed before adding more.

5. In a separate pan, sauté sliced mushrooms until browned and tender.

6. Once the rice is creamy and cooked to al dente, stir in the sautéed mushrooms and baby spinach leaves.

7. Remove from heat and stir in grated Parmesan cheese. Season with salt and pepper to taste.

8. Garnish with fresh parsley before serving.

Lemon Garlic Shrimp Pasta

Ingredients:

- 8 ounces whole wheat spaghetti

- 1 pound large shrimp, peeled and deveined

- 2 tablespoons olive oil

- 4 cloves garlic, minced

- Zest and juice of 1 lemon

- 1/4 cup chopped fresh parsley

- Salt and pepper to taste

- Grated Parmesan cheese for serving

Prep Time: 10 mins

Cooking Time: 15 mins

Total Time: 25 mins

Servings: 4

Nutrition Facts (per serving):

- 350 Calories

- Fat 10g

- Saturated fat 2g

- Cholesterol 160mg

- Sodium 260mg

- Carbohydrate 40g

- Protein 30g

- Fiber 6g

Instructions:

1. Cook whole wheat spaghetti according to package instructions until al dente. Drain and set aside.

2. In a large skillet, heat olive oil over medium heat. Add minced garlic and cook until fragrant, about 1-2 minutes.

3. Add peeled and deveined shrimp to the skillet and cook until pink and opaque, about 2-3 minutes per side.

4. Stir in lemon zest, lemon juice, chopped fresh parsley, salt, and pepper.

5. Add cooked spaghetti to the skillet and toss well to coat the pasta evenly with the shrimp and garlic-lemon sauce.

6. Serve hot, garnished with grated Parmesan cheese.

Honey Mustard Glazed Salmon

Ingredients:

- 4 salmon fillets
- 2 tablespoons Dijon mustard
- 2 tablespoons honey
- 1 tablespoon olive oil
- 2 cloves garlic, minced
- Salt and pepper to taste
- Fresh lemon wedges for serving
- Fresh dill for garnish

Prep Time: 10 mins

Cooking Time: 15 mins

Total Time: 25 mins

Servings: 4

Nutrition Facts (per serving):

- 280 Calories
- Fat 15g
- Saturated fat 3g
- Cholesterol 80mg
- Sodium 280mg

- Carbohydrate 10g

- Protein 25g

Instructions:

1. Preheat oven to 375°F (190°C).

2. In a small bowl, whisk together Dijon mustard, honey, olive oil, minced garlic, salt, and pepper.

3. Place salmon fillets on a baking sheet lined with parchment paper.

4. Brush honey mustard glaze evenly over the tops of the salmon fillets.

5. Bake in the preheated oven for 12-15 minutes, or until salmon flakes easily with a fork and reaches an internal temperature of 145°F (63°C).

6. Remove from oven and let rest for a few minutes before serving.

7. Serve hot, garnished with fresh dill and lemon wedges.

Vegetable and Lentil Curry

Ingredients:

- 1 cup dried green or brown lentils, rinsed

- 4 cups vegetable broth

- 1 cup diced carrots

- 1 cup diced celery

- 1 cup diced onions

- 2 cloves garlic, minced

- 1 teaspoon dried thyme

- 1 teaspoon dried oregano

- 1 tablespoon curry powder

- Salt and pepper to taste

- 2 tablespoons olive oil

Prep Time: 10 mins

Cooking Time: 30 mins

Total Time: 40 mins

Servings: 4

Nutrition Facts (per serving):

- 220 Calories

- Fat 6g

- Saturated fat 1g

- Cholesterol 0mg

- Sodium 480mg

- Carbohydrate 32g

- Protein 12g

- Fiber 12g

Instructions:

1. In a large pot, heat olive oil over medium heat.

2. Add diced onions, carrots, and celery to the pot. Cook until vegetables are softened, about 5-7 minutes.

3. Add minced garlic, dried thyme, dried oregano, and curry powder to the pot. Cook for an additional 1-2 minutes until fragrant.

4. Pour vegetable broth into the pot and bring to a simmer.

5. Add rinsed lentils to the pot and stir well to combine.

6. Cover the pot and simmer for 20-25 minutes until lentils are tender.

7. Season with salt and pepper to taste.

8. Serve hot as a comforting and nutritious dinner option.

SNACKS AND DESSERT RECIPES

Apple Cinnamon Oatmeal Muffins

Ingredients:

- 1 cup rolled oats
- 1 cup whole wheat flour
- 1 teaspoon baking powder
- 1/2 teaspoon baking soda
- 1/2 teaspoon ground cinnamon
- 1/4 teaspoon salt
- 2 large eggs
- 1/4 cup honey or maple syrup
- 1/4 cup unsweetened applesauce
- 1/4 cup milk of choice
- 1 teaspoon vanilla extract
- 1 cup diced apples

Prep Time: 10 mins

Cooking Time: 20 mins

Total Time: 30 mins

Servings: 12

Nutrition Facts (per serving):

- 120 Calories
- Fat 2g
- Saturated fat 0.5g

- Cholesterol 30mg

- Sodium 150mg

- Carbohydrate 22g

- Protein 4g

- Fiber 2g

Instructions:

1. Preheat oven to 350°F (175°C). Grease or line a muffin tin with paper liners.

2. In a large bowl, combine rolled oats, whole wheat flour, baking powder, baking soda, cinnamon, and salt.

3. In another bowl, whisk together eggs, honey or maple syrup, applesauce, milk, and vanilla extract until well combined.

4. Pour wet ingredients into dry ingredients and mix until just combined.

5. Fold in diced apples.

6. Divide batter evenly among muffin cups, filling each about 3/4 full.

7. Bake for 18-20 minutes, or until a toothpick inserted into the centre comes out clean.

8. Allow muffins to cool in the pan for 5 minutes before transferring to a wire rack to cool completely.

Greek Yogurt Parfait

Ingredients:

- 1 cup Greek yogurt

- 1/2 cup granola

- 1/2 cup mixed berries (strawberries, blueberries, raspberries)

- 1 tablespoon honey (optional)

- Fresh mint leaves for garnish

Prep Time: 5 mins

Total Time: 5 mins

Servings: 1

Nutrition Facts (per serving):

- 250 Calories

- Fat 5g

- Saturated fat 1g

- Cholesterol 5mg

- Sodium 50mg

- Carbohydrate 40g

- Protein 15g

- Fiber 5g

Instructions:

1. In a glass or serving bowl, layer Greek yogurt, granola, and mixed berries.

2. Drizzle honey over the top, if desired.

3. Garnish with fresh mint leaves.

4. Serve immediately as a refreshing and nutritious snack or dessert option.

Avocado Chocolate Pudding

Ingredients:

- 2 ripe avocados
- 1/4 cup cocoa powder
- 1/4 cup honey or maple syrup
- 1 teaspoon vanilla extract
- Pinch of salt
- 1/4 cup almond milk (or any milk of choice)
- Fresh berries for garnish

Prep Time: 10 mins

Total Time: 10 mins

Servings: 4

Nutrition Facts (per serving):

- 200 Calories
- Fat 14g
- Saturated fat 2g
- Cholesterol 0mg
- Sodium 50mg
- Carbohydrate 22g
- Protein 3g
- Fiber 6g

Instructions:

1. Scoop out the flesh of the ripe avocados and place them in a blender or food processor.

2. Add cocoa powder, honey or maple syrup, vanilla extract, salt, and almond milk to the blender.

3. Blend until smooth and creamy, scraping down the sides of the blender as needed.

4. Divide the chocolate avocado pudding into serving bowls.

5. Chill in the refrigerator for at least 30 minutes before serving.

6. Garnish with fresh berries before serving.

Banana Almond Butter Energy Bites

Ingredients:

- 1 ripe banana, mashed

- 1/2 cup rolled oats

- 1/4 cup almond butter

- 2 tablespoons honey

- 1/4 teaspoon ground cinnamon

- 1/4 cup chopped almonds

- 1/4 cup shredded coconut (optional)

Prep Time: 10 mins

Total Time: 10 mins

Servings: 12

Nutrition Facts (per serving, 2 energy bites):

- 120 Calories
- Fat 7g
- Saturated fat 1g
- Cholesterol 0mg
- Sodium 5mg
- Carbohydrate 12g
- Protein 3g
- Fiber 2g

Instructions:

1. In a mixing bowl, combine mashed banana, rolled oats, almond butter, honey, and ground cinnamon.
2. Stir in chopped almonds and shredded coconut, if using.
3. Roll the mixture into small balls using your hands.
4. Place energy bites on a baking sheet lined with parchment paper.
5. Chill in the refrigerator for at least 30 minutes before serving.
6. Store leftovers in an airtight container in the refrigerator for up to one week.

Chia Seed Pudding

Ingredients:

- 1/4 cup chia seeds
- 1 cup almond milk (or any milk of choice)

- 1 tablespoon honey or maple syrup

- 1/2 teaspoon vanilla extract

- Fresh fruit for topping (e.g., berries, sliced banana)

Prep Time: 5 mins

Total Time: 4 hours 5 mins (includes chilling time)

Servings: 2

Nutrition Facts (per serving):

- 120 Calories

- Fat 6g

- Saturated fat 0.5g

- Cholesterol 0mg

- Sodium 80mg

- Carbohydrate 13g

- Protein 4g

- Fiber 8g

Instructions:

1. In a bowl, whisk together chia seeds, almond milk, honey or maple syrup, and vanilla extract.

2. Cover the bowl and refrigerate for at least 4 hours or overnight, stirring occasionally.

3. Once the chia seed pudding has thickened to your desired consistency, divide it into serving cups.

4. Top with fresh fruit before serving.

5. Enjoy chilled as a healthy and filling snack or dessert option.

Sweet Potato Toast with Almond Butter and Banana

Ingredients:

- 1 medium sweet potato, sliced into 1/4-inch thick rounds

- 2 tablespoons almond butter

- 1 ripe banana, thinly sliced

- 1 tablespoon honey (optional)

- Pinch of cinnamon (optional)

Prep Time: 5 mins Cooking Time: 10 mins Total Time: 15 mins Servings: 2

Nutrition Facts (per serving):

- 180 Calories

- Fat 8g

- Saturated fat 1g

- Cholesterol 0mg

- Sodium 50mg

- Carbohydrate 26g

- Protein 4g

- Fiber 4g

Instructions:

1. Preheat oven to 400°F (200°C). Place sweet potato slices on a baking sheet lined with parchment paper.

2. Bake sweet potato slices for 10-15 minutes, or until tender.

3. Remove sweet potato slices from the oven and let cool slightly.

4. Spread almond butter on each sweet potato slice.

5. Top with thinly sliced banana.

6. Drizzle with honey and sprinkle with cinnamon, if desired.

7. Serve immediately as a delicious and nutritious snack.

Mixed Berry Chia Jam

Ingredients:

- 2 cups mixed berries (strawberries, blueberries, raspberries)

- 2 tablespoons chia seeds

- 1 tablespoon honey or maple syrup

- 1/2 teaspoon vanilla extract

Prep Time: 5 mins

Cooking Time: 10 mins

Total Time: 15 mins

Servings: 8

Nutrition Facts (per serving):

- 40 Calories

- Fat 1g

- Saturated fat 0g

- Cholesterol 0mg

- Sodium 0mg

- Carbohydrate 8g

- Protein 1g

- Fiber 3g

Instructions:

1. In a saucepan, combine mixed berries and honey or maple syrup.

2. Cook over medium heat, stirring occasionally, until berries begin to break down and release their juices, about 5-7 minutes.

3. Mash the berries with a fork or potato masher to desired consistency.

4. Stir in chia seeds and vanilla extract.

5. Continue to cook for an additional 5 minutes, stirring frequently, until the jam thickens.

6. Remove from heat and let cool completely.

7. Transfer the chia jam to a jar and store in the refrigerator for up to one week.

8. Enjoy spread on whole grain toast, yogurt, or oatmeal.

Frozen Yogurt Bark

Ingredients:

- 2 cups Greek yogurt

- 2 tablespoons honey or maple syrup

- 1/2 cup mixed berries (strawberries, blueberries, raspberries)

- 1/4 cup chopped nuts (almonds, walnuts, pecans)

- 2 tablespoons shredded coconut

Prep Time: 5 mins

Freezing Time: 2 hours

Total Time: 2 hours 5 mins

Servings: 8

Nutrition Facts (per serving):

- 80 Calories

- Fat 3g

- Saturated fat 1g

- Cholesterol 0mg

- Sodium 20mg

- Carbohydrate 9g

- Protein 5g

- Fiber 1g

Instructions:

1. Line a baking sheet with parchment paper.

2. In a bowl, mix together Greek yogurt and honey or maple syrup until well combined.

3. Spread the yogurt mixture evenly onto the prepared baking sheet.

4. Sprinkle mixed berries, chopped nuts, and shredded coconut over the yogurt mixture.

5. Place the baking sheet in the freezer and freeze for at least 2 hours, or until the yogurt bark is firm.

6. Once frozen, break the yogurt bark into pieces.

7. Serve immediately as a refreshing and nutritious snack.

Chocolate Banana Nice Cream

Ingredients:

- 3 ripe bananas, sliced and frozen
- 2 tablespoons cocoa powder
- 1 tablespoon honey or maple syrup
- 1/4 cup almond milk (or any milk of choice)
- 1/4 teaspoon vanilla extract
- Dark chocolate chips for topping (optional)

Prep Time: 5 mins

Freezing Time: 2 hours

Total Time: 2 hours 5 mins

Servings: 2

Nutrition Facts (per serving):

- 180 Calories
- Fat 2g
- Saturated fat 1g
- Cholesterol 0mg
- Sodium 10mg
- Carbohydrate 45g
- Protein 3g
- Fiber 6g

Instructions:

1. Place frozen banana slices in a blender or food processor.

2. Add cocoa powder, honey or maple syrup, almond milk, and vanilla extract to the blender.

3. Blend until smooth and creamy, scraping down the sides of the blender as needed.

4. Transfer the chocolate banana nice cream to a freezer-safe container.

5. Freeze for at least 2 hours, or until firm.

6. Serve scoops of chocolate banana nice cream topped with dark chocolate chips, if desired.

No-Bake Energy Bites

Ingredients:

- 1 cup rolled oats

- 1/2 cup almond butter

- 1/4 cup honey or maple syrup

- 1/4 cup unsweetened shredded coconut

- 1/4 cup mini chocolate chips

- 1 teaspoon vanilla extract

- Pinch of salt

Prep Time: 10 mins

Total Time: 10 mins

Servings: 12

Nutrition Facts (per serving, 2 energy bites):

- 160 Calories

- Fat 9g

- Saturated fat 2g

- Cholesterol 0mg

- Sodium 20mg

- Carbohydrate 16g

- Protein 4g

- Fiber 2g

Instructions:

1. In a mixing bowl, combine rolled oats, almond butter, honey or maple syrup, shredded coconut, mini chocolate chips, vanilla extract, and a pinch of salt.

2. Stir until well combined.

3. Roll the mixture into small balls using your hands.

4. Place energy bites on a baking sheet lined with parchment paper.

5. Chill in the refrigerator for at least 30 minutes before serving.

6. Store leftovers in an airtight container in the refrigerator for up to one week.

BEVERAGES RECIPES

Green Smoothie

Ingredients:

- 1 cup spinach leaves
- 1/2 cup kale leaves
- 1/2 cup cucumber, chopped
- 1/2 banana, frozen
- 1/2 cup pineapple chunks, frozen
- 1/2 cup unsweetened almond milk
- 1/2 cup Greek yogurt
- 1 tablespoon honey or maple syrup (optional)
- Ice cubes (optional)

Prep Time: 5 mins

Total Time: 5 mins

Servings: 2

Nutrition Facts (per serving):

- 100 Calories
- Fat 2g
- Saturated fat 0.5g
- Cholesterol 0mg

- Sodium 80mg

- Carbohydrate 20g

- Protein 5g

- Fiber 4g

Instructions:

1. Place spinach, kale, cucumber, banana, pineapple, almond milk, Greek yogurt, and honey or maple syrup (if using) in a blender.

2. Blend until smooth and creamy.

3. Add ice cubes if desired for a colder consistency.

4. Pour into glasses and serve immediately as a refreshing and nutrient-packed beverage.

Turmeric Latte

Ingredients:

- 1 cup unsweetened almond milk

- 1 teaspoon ground turmeric

- 1/2 teaspoon ground cinnamon

- 1/4 teaspoon ground ginger

- 1/4 teaspoon ground nutmeg

- 1 tablespoon honey or maple syrup (optional)

- Pinch of black pepper

Prep Time: 5 mins

Cooking Time: 5 mins

Total Time: 10 mins

Servings: 1

Nutrition Facts (per serving):

- 60 Calories

- Fat 2g

- Saturated fat 0g

- Cholesterol 0mg

- Sodium 160mg

- Carbohydrate 10g

- Protein 1g

- Fiber 2g

Instructions:

1. In a small saucepan, heat almond milk over medium heat until hot but not boiling.

2. Whisk in ground turmeric, ground cinnamon, ground ginger, ground nutmeg, honey or maple syrup (if using), and a pinch of black pepper.

3. Continue to whisk until well combined and heated through.

4. Pour turmeric latte into a mug and serve immediately, optionally garnishing with a sprinkle of ground cinnamon on top.

Berry Blast Smoothie

Ingredients:

- 1/2 cup mixed berries (strawberries, blueberries, raspberries)

- 1/2 banana, frozen

- 1/2 cup plain Greek yogurt

- 1/2 cup unsweetened almond milk

- 1 tablespoon chia seeds

- 1 tablespoon honey or maple syrup (optional)

- Ice cubes (optional)

Prep Time: 5 mins

Total Time: 5 mins

Servings: 1

Nutrition Facts (per serving):

- 150 Calories

- Fat 4g

- Saturated fat 0.5g

- Cholesterol 0mg

- Sodium 60mg

- Carbohydrate 23g

- Protein 9g

- Fiber 5g

Instructions:

1. Place mixed berries, banana, Greek yogurt, almond milk, chia seeds, and honey or maple syrup (if using) in a blender.

2. Blend until smooth and creamy.

3. Add ice cubes if desired for a colder consistency.

4. Pour into a glass and serve immediately as a delicious and nutritious beverage option.

Coconut Water Refresher

Ingredients:

- 1 cup coconut water

- 1/2 cup pineapple juice

- 1/4 cup lime juice

- 1 tablespoon honey or maple syrup (optional)

- Mint leaves for garnish (optional)

Prep Time: 5 mins

Total Time: 5 mins

Servings: 1

Nutrition Facts (per serving):

- 90 Calories

- Fat 0g

- Saturated fat 0g

- Cholesterol 0mg

- Sodium 35mg

- Carbohydrate 23g

- Protein 0g

- Fiber 0g

Instructions:

1. In a glass, combine coconut water, pineapple juice, lime juice, and honey or maple syrup (if using).

2. Stir until well combined.

3. Garnish with fresh mint leaves, if desired.

4. Serve immediately over ice as a hydrating and refreshing beverage option.

Iced Matcha Latte

Ingredients:

- 1 teaspoon matcha powder

- 1 tablespoon hot water

- 1 cup unsweetened almond milk

- 1 tablespoon honey or maple syrup (optional)

- Ice cubes

Prep Time: 5 mins

Total Time: 5 mins

Servings: 1

Nutrition Facts (per serving):

- 60 Calories

- Fat 2g

- Saturated fat 0g

- Cholesterol 0mg

- Sodium 160mg

- Carbohydrate 10g

- Protein 1g

- Fiber 1g

Instructions:

1. In a small bowl, whisk matcha powder with hot water until smooth and dissolved.

2. In a glass, combine matcha mixture, almond milk, and honey or maple syrup (if using).

3. Stir until well combined.

4. Add ice cubes to the glass.

5. Serve immediately as a refreshing and energizing beverage option.

Golden Milk

Ingredients:

- 1 cup unsweetened almond milk

- 1 teaspoon ground turmeric

- 1/2 teaspoon ground cinnamon

- 1/4 teaspoon ground ginger

- Pinch of ground black pepper

- 1 tablespoon honey or maple syrup (optional)

Prep Time: 5 mins

Cooking Time: 5 mins

Total Time: 10 mins

Servings: 1

Nutrition Facts (per serving):

- 60 Calories

- Fat 2g

- Saturated fat 0g

- Cholesterol 0mg

- Sodium 160mg

- Carbohydrate 10g

- Protein 1g

- Fiber 1g

Instructions:

1. In a small saucepan, heat almond milk over medium heat until hot but not boiling.

2. Whisk in ground turmeric, ground cinnamon, ground ginger, and a pinch of black pepper.

3. Continue to whisk until well combined and heated through.

4. Add honey or maple syrup (if using) and stir until dissolved.

5. Pour golden milk into a mug and serve immediately as a soothing and warming beverage.

Mango Lassi

Ingredients:

- 1 ripe mango, peeled and diced

- 1/2 cup plain Greek yogurt

- 1/2 cup unsweetened almond milk

- 1 tablespoon honey or maple syrup (optional)

- 1/4 teaspoon ground cardamom

- Ice cubes

Prep Time: 5 mins

Total Time: 5 mins

Servings: 1

Nutrition Facts (per serving):

- 180 Calories

- Fat 2g

- Saturated fat 0g

- Cholesterol 0mg

- Sodium 50mg

- Carbohydrate 37g

- Protein 8g

- Fiber 3g

Instructions:

1. Place diced mango, Greek yogurt, almond milk, honey or maple syrup (if using), and ground cardamom in a blender.

2. Blend until smooth and creamy.

3. Add ice cubes for a colder consistency, if desired, and blend again until smooth.

4. Pour mango lassi into a glass and serve immediately as a refreshing and tropical beverage.

Berry Hibiscus Iced Tea

Ingredients:

- 2 hibiscus tea bags

- 2 cups boiling water

- 1/2 cup mixed berries (strawberries, blueberries, raspberries)

- 1 tablespoon honey or maple syrup (optional)

- Fresh lemon slices for garnish (optional)

- Ice cubes

Prep Time: 5 mins

Cooking Time: 5 mins

Total Time: 10 mins

Servings: 2

Nutrition Facts (per serving):

- 20 Calories

- Fat 0g

- Saturated fat 0g

- Cholesterol 0mg

- Sodium 5mg

- Carbohydrate 5g

- Protein 0g

- Fiber 1g

Instructions:

1. Place hibiscus tea bags in a heatproof pitcher.

2. Pour boiling water over the tea bags and let steep for 5 minutes.

3. Remove tea bags and discard.

4. Add mixed berries and honey or maple syrup (if using) to the pitcher.

5. Stir until honey or maple syrup is dissolved and the berries are slightly mashed.

6. Let the tea cool to room temperature, then refrigerate until chilled.

7. Serve over ice with fresh lemon slices for garnish, if desired.

Pineapple Coconut Water Smoothie

Ingredients:

- 1 cup coconut water

- 1 cup frozen pineapple chunks

- 1/2 banana, frozen

- 1/2 cup plain Greek yogurt

- 1 tablespoon honey or maple syrup (optional)

- Ice cubes

Prep Time: 5 mins

Total Time: 5 mins

Servings: 1

Nutrition Facts (per serving):

- 150 Calories

- Fat 1g

- Saturated fat 0g

- Cholesterol 0mg

- Sodium 100mg

- Carbohydrate 30g

- Protein 8g

- Fiber 2g

Instructions:

1. Place coconut water, frozen pineapple chunks, frozen banana, Greek yogurt, and honey or maple syrup (if using) in a blender.

2. Blend until smooth and creamy.

3. Add ice cubes for a colder consistency, if desired, and blend again until smooth.

4. Pour pineapple coconut water smoothie into a glass and serve immediately as a tropical and hydrating beverage.

Cucumber Mint Infused Water

Ingredients:

- 4 cups water

- 1 cucumber, thinly sliced

- 1/4 cup fresh mint leaves

- Ice cubes

Prep Time: 5 mins

Total Time: 5 mins

Servings: 4

Nutrition Facts (per serving):

- 0 Calories

- Fat 0g

- Saturated fat 0g

- Cholesterol 0mg

- Sodium 0mg

- Carbohydrate 0g

- Protein 0g

- Fiber 0g

Instructions:

1. In a pitcher, combine water, sliced cucumber, and fresh mint leaves.

2. Stir gently to combine.

3. Refrigerate for at least 1 hour to allow the flavors to infuse.

4. Serve cucumber mint infused water over ice for a refreshing and hydrating beverage option.

21 DAY MEAL PLAN

Day 1:

- ***Breakfast:*** Green Smoothie

- ***Lunch:*** Golden Milk

- ***Dinner:*** Berry Hibiscus Iced Tea

Day 2:

- ***Breakfast:*** Mango Lassi

- ***Lunch:*** Cucumber Mint Infused Water

- ***Dinner:*** Pineapple Coconut Water Smoothie

Day 3:

- ***Breakfast:*** Turmeric Latte

- ***Lunch:*** Berry Blast Smoothie

- ***Dinner:*** Coconut Water Refresher

Day 4:

- ***Breakfast:*** Iced Matcha Latte

- ***Lunch:*** Pineapple Coconut Water Smoothie

- ***Dinner:*** Golden Milk

Day 5:

- ***Breakfast:*** Berry Hibiscus Iced Tea

- ***Lunch:*** Green Smoothie

- *Dinner:* Mango Lassi

Day 6:

- *Breakfast:* Coconut Water Refresher

- *Lunch:* Turmeric Latte

- *Dinner:* Berry Blast Smoothie

Day 7:

- *Breakfast:* Cucumber Mint Infused Water

- *Lunch:* Golden Milk

- *Dinner:* Iced Matcha Latte

Day 8:

- *Breakfast:* Pineapple Coconut Water Smoothie

- *Lunch:* Berry Hibiscus Iced Tea

- *Dinner:* Green Smoothie

Day 9:

- *Breakfast:* Mango Lassi

- *Lunch:* Coconut Water Refresher

- *Dinner:* Turmeric Latte

Day 10:

- *Breakfast:* Berry Blast Smoothie

- *Lunch:* Iced Matcha Latte

- *Dinner:* Cucumber Mint Infused Water

Day 11:

- *Breakfast:* Golden Milk

- *Lunch:* Pineapple Coconut Water Smoothie

- *Dinner:* Berry Hibiscus Iced Tea

Day 12:

- *Breakfast:* Berry Blast Smoothie

- *Lunch:* Coconut Water Refresher

- *Dinner:* Turmeric Latte

Day 13:

- *Breakfast:* Green Smoothie

- *Lunch:* Iced Matcha Latte

- *Dinner:* Cucumber Mint Infused Water

Day 14:

- *Breakfast*: Mango Lassi

- *Lunch:* Berry Hibiscus Iced Tea

- *Dinner:* Golden Milk

Day 15:

- *Breakfast:* Coconut Water Refresher

- *Lunch:* Turmeric Latte

- *Dinner:* Berry Blast Smoothie

Day 16:

- *Breakfast:* Pineapple Coconut Water Smoothie

- *Lunch:* Green Smoothie

- *Dinner:* Mango Lassi

Day 17:

- *Breakfast:* Iced Matcha Latte

- *Lunch:* Cucumber Mint Infused Water

- *Dinner:* Golden Milk

Day 18:

- *Breakfast:* Berry Hibiscus Iced Tea

- *Lunch:* Coconut Water Refresher

- *Dinner:* Turmeric Latte

Day 19:

- *Breakfast:* Berry Blast Smoothie

- *Lunch:* Pineapple Coconut Water Smoothie

- *Dinner:* Green Smoothie

Day 20:

- *Breakfast:* Mango Lassi

- *Lunch:* Golden Milk

- ***Dinner:*** Cucumber Mint Infused Water

Day 21:

- ***Breakfast:*** Iced Matcha Latte

- ***Lunch:*** Berry Hibiscus Iced Tea

- ***Dinner:*** Coconut Water Refresher

CONCLUSION

In conclusion, embarking on the journey of adopting the EPI Diet Cookbook and Food List for Beginners can be a transformative experience for individuals managing exocrine pancreatic insufficiency (EPI). Through our exploration of various meal plans and recipes, we've highlighted the importance of incorporating nutrient-dense foods while being mindful of ingredients that may exacerbate EPI symptoms.

From the vibrant array of breakfast smoothies to the soothing warmth of turmeric lattes, our meal plans offer a diverse range of flavourful and nourishing options. Each recipe is thoughtfully crafted to prioritize ingredients that support digestive health and minimize discomfort associated with EPI. By focusing on whole foods rich in protein, healthy fats, vitamins, and minerals, individuals can optimize their nutritional intake while managing EPI symptoms effectively

Furthermore, our exploration of beverages has underscored the significance of hydration and the role of refreshing drinks in maintaining overall well-being. From hydrating coconut water smoothies to antioxidant-rich berry hibiscus iced tea, these beverages offer a delicious way to stay hydrated while enjoying a variety of flavours.

As we conclude our discussion, it's important to recognize that adopting the EPI Diet Cookbook and Food List for Beginners is not just about managing symptoms—it's about embracing a lifestyle centred around nourishment and wellness. By incorporating these recipes into your daily routine, you're not only supporting your digestive health but also cultivating a deeper connection with the food you consume.

www.ingramcontent.com/pod-product-compliance
Lightning Source LLC
Chambersburg PA
CBHW071221260726